NO POT, NO WINDOW
Or
"How I Changed My Life from Sour Lemons to Sweet Lemonade"

NO POT, NO WINDOW

OR

"HOW I CHANGED MY LIFE FROM SOUR LEMONS TO SWEET LEMONADE"

Mary King, Lt., USN, Retired

With a Contribution from my sister,

Anne Evans

Library of Congress Control Number:		2010907302
ISBN:	Hardcover	978-1-4535-0630-1
	Softcover	978-1-4535-0629-5
	E-book	978-1-4535-0631-8

To order additional copies of this book, contact:
Xlibris Corporation
1-888-795-4274
www.Xlibris.com
Orders@Xlibris.com
81316

CONTENTS

DEDICATION

This book is dedicated to my deceased mother who did her best with her limited capabilities and to my daughter, Dannielle, who endured many hardships as a dependent of an active duty military mom.

I also want to acknowledge all the veterans who proudly serve or have served our country especially the Viet Nam Veterans who were so unappreciated.

Finally, since I am a 26 year survivor, I would be remiss if I did not pay tribute to the brave warriors who have battled breast cancer. Sadly, the fight continues since there is still no cure for this deadly disease.

CHAPTER 1

Introduction

If you are under 40 years of age, you probably don't have a clue what the expression "no pot, no window" means. It is a southern expression which I acquired from my late maternal grandmother who was a young woman during the Great Depression of 1929. It means no pot to pee in and no window to throw it out. In other words, you are very poor, have virtually nothing and there is little chance of changing your pathetic circumstances. Now, add Texas white trash to the mix and that is the description of the family to whom I was born. What is to follow is a true story about my life and how I was finally successful in scratching and clawing my way out of the "no pot, no window" syndrome as well as surviving Stage II breast cancer diagnosed when I was only 32 years old. I believe poverty, lack of education, a negative home environment, alcohol and/or drug abuse, bad judgment, a single parent home, disease/illness, and sometimes just plain bad luck keeps the cycle of "no pot, no window" perpetuating generation after generation. I hope this novel serves as a motivator and an inspiration to the thousands of people with similar circumstances that think they have no options in life. We all have options since our lives are not predestined. Anything in life is possible if you want it bad enough and refuse to accept the life of "no pot, no window". We are all capable of changing our lives from sour lemons to sweet lemonade.

CHAPTER 2

The Early Years (Age 5-9)

I was born and spent my first nine years of life in East Texas, Marshall, to be exact. I have two sisters, Anne, four years older and Betty, about one and a half years younger. Neither of my parents graduated from school. My father completed the fifth grade and my mother made it through the eighth grade. My parents met and subsequently married shortly after my father's discharge from the Army at the end of World War II. I was born in 1951, so this is where the story begins.

From as early as I can remember, my father worked for the railroad in Marshall and my mother was as we say now, a stay at home mom. This was the appropriate lifestyle in the '50's and early '60's. The man was the breadwinner and the woman was in charge of the kids and the house. Life is so different today.

To the best of my memory, the first six or seven years of my life were good. Our family was lower middle class and wanted for little of nothing. My father was making a decent salary at the railroad and when I was four or five he bought a small, three bedroom, one bath house on East Fannin Street. The house had a screened in back porch which my father later converted into another bedroom, so technically I guess you say our house had four bedrooms. Anne moved into the converted fourth bedroom when she was nine or ten which was good because Betty and I slept in the bedroom next to it. Mom and Dad had the two front bedrooms and the three of us kids had the two rear bedrooms. The bathroom was in the middle of the house between the two sets of bedrooms. This is significant because when mom and dad argued the distance between their bedroom(s) and ours acted as a buffer and drowned out some of the noise. The first vehicle I remember my father driving was a 1955 brown and white Ford Fairlane. We were one of the lucky families who had a television set shortly after they came on the market. In the mid fifties, television broadcasting didn't start until early afternoon, there were only three or four black and white channels, and it went off the air shortly after the ten o'clock news. My favorite programs were the "Mickey Mouse Club"," I Love Lucy", "Gunsmoke", and "Rawhide". My parents didn't go out much so we all generally stayed at home, enjoyed each others company and watched our fancy television. Occasionally, my father invited some of his married co-workers over for a spin at dominos. When I was around eight years old the bottom fell out. The "Cleaver" house was no more.

My father, who was a fourth Cherokee Indian, started drinking heavily and wouldn't stop. He always drank some but not like this and when he drank he got mean. His constant drinking interfered with his job at the railroad, so he stopped going to work. My parents were arguing all the time now and there were no more family nights in front of the television. No more domino parties either. Just one drunken argument after another. Of course, he eventually lost his good paying job at the railroad and there was no money coming in to pay the bills and buy groceries. After 12 years on the job, the railroad let him go with a very small severance check. And that was that. No money! A family of five can't live without money for very long.

After my father lost his job, he quit coming home or came home in the middle of the night drunk. He woke all of us up with his drunken antics and the arguing between him and my mother started again just like it did virtually every night now. I remember wishing that I would become very sick or even die and that would bring them closer and life would return to normal. I would hold my breath for as long as I could and imagine me in a coffin. I guess that was my way of crying for help.

The arguing between my parents eventually turned to physical abuse and violence. Anne, Betty and I started hiding, usually under our beds. One night, when the noise got so loud, I got out of bed and snuck into the living room where my parents were arguing and was horrified by what I saw. My father was holding a shotgun to my mother's head and yelling he was going to blow her brains out. In the late '50's, there was no such thing as domestic violence or domestic abuse. The husband ruled the house and the house was his castle. The wife was considered property of the man and therefore, this was a private family matter. In other words, there was no point calling the police. After witnessing that episode, I yelled and ran back to bed. The violence ended for the night but resumed again a few nights later. Eventually, my father quit coming home all together. He later claimed he was out of town looking for work.

For the next year or so, my parents' marriage was off and on but technically they were separated. My father moved to Houston for work and we stayed in the house on Fannin Street. I remember my mother cried a lot and went to the doctor for depression. Apparently, the doctor recommended she start smoking to help calm her nerves and he gave her something to help her sleep. Mom bought a couple of packs of Winstons and attempted to start smoking. This was quite humorous. She would light the cigarette, hold it way out in front of her because she didn't like the smoke and puff on it without inhaling. She gave up trying to smoke after a couple of weeks. Since my father was only coming home maybe one weekend a month, I have no idea how the bills were getting paid. Mom just went to bed early and cried.

Over the next year or so, my parents tried a short reconciliation. They either bought or rented a lake house on Caddo Lake not far from my paternal grandparents in Karnack and we moved there for the summer. I don't remember anybody working that summer. It was all about my father drinking, fishing, frog gigging, and listening to Hank Williams "Your Cheatin Heart". Mom liked Patsy Cline, particularly her song "Crazy". It's one of my favorites also. I don't remember what Anne did that summer but my parents bought Betty and me a Candyland board game and we entertained ourselves with it in our bedroom while Mom and Dad partied until the wee hours of the morning in the living room. After a couple of months at the lake house it started to rain. It rained for what seemed like weeks and the lake house flooded even though it was on stilts raised about eight feet off the ground. We managed to retrieve a few of our belongings and abandoned the lake house in our fishing boat. Since we now had nowhere to live, the entire family moved into my paternal grandparent's small home for a couple of weeks then my father packed up and went back to Houston. Their marriage was truly over now.

Mom, Anne, Betty and I moved back into the house on Fannin Street and life moved on. Mother, who only had an eighth grade education, managed to get a job as a cashier at the local grocery store and eventually could afford to buy a car. While she was at work,

Anne was in charge of the house which included Betty and me. Anne was only eleven or twelve years old and far too young for this responsibility. Actually, she resented it and took it out on Betty and me. She would pull us around the house by our hair in order to make us mind. Things did not go well. Anne didn't know how to cook so unless mother cooked something before she left for work or a night on the town, we didn't eat. Betty and I got used to fending for ourselves—begging food from neighbors or making mayonnaise sandwiches. When my father was living at home we always had deer meat, squirrel, rabbit, or fish to eat since he was a gamesman. Mother's usual meal was pressure cooker spaghetti which was mush you had to pry out of the pan or pig's brains and eggs which tasted absolutely horrible. Anne had a hole in the floor where she sat at the table and was able to poke most of her pig's brains and eggs down the hole. Betty and I weren't so lucky because we didn't have a hole to poke that mess down and had to eat at least three quarters of what was on our plate before we could leave the table. Anne, Betty and I went to bed hungry a lot of nights because we couldn't stand eating her cooking. I had just started the fourth grade and had no clothes to start school except hand-me downs from Anne and one of my cousins. I was always a little chunky, so nothing fit. They either looked like I had been poured into them or they were going to fall off of me. Betty was easier to dress since she was tall and slim. It is a lot easier to take up clothes than let them out.

Mom was gone most of the time now and when she was home she didn't want to spend time with us kids. Anne was old enough to go out on her own to a friend's house or visit a neighbor. Betty and I didn't have that option because we were too young. Mother used to lock the three of us out of the house for hours in the afternoon while she slept. We got water out of a water hose in the yard but didn't have bathroom facilities. I remember beating on the screen door telling mom that I had to go to the bathroom but she never got up and let me in the house. Therefore, I had the option of peeing in the yard or going down the street to my great aunt Ollie's house to use the bathroom. I really don't know how we all survived that year. As far as I know, my father never made any attempt to help us financially. The few times I saw him that year were a disaster—he had moved on with his life so to speak. He was an alcoholic, living with another woman, and neither one of them were working more than one or two days a week. Things had gone from bad to worse so mom called Anne, Betty and I into the kitchen one night and told us we were going to go live with her parents, Big Momma and Little Daddy for awhile. Mom said she couldn't support us or take care of us and work. She also said it was either living with her parents or be put up for adoption. Now I really felt abandoned—first no father and now no mother. She said we would be orphans. Maybe it would have been better for the three of us kids if she had made us wards of the state because we didn't really have parents from this point on. My mother and father should have never had children because Anne, Betty and I were the biggest losers in their marriage. We were neglected, abandoned, and abused during our childhood which subsequently scarred all three of us for life. Honestly, I think mother was looking for an easy way out by finding another husband to take care of her financially and Anne, Betty and I were just in the way. She had recently started dating her supervisor from the grocery store but a woman with three clinging kids wasn't exactly appealing to most men. My mother was married eight or nine times and was codependent. Even though she eventually obtained her G.E.D., she didn't want to work and be self sufficient. And most of all, she didn't want to support three kids on her own. My mother was always looking for the right frog to kiss.

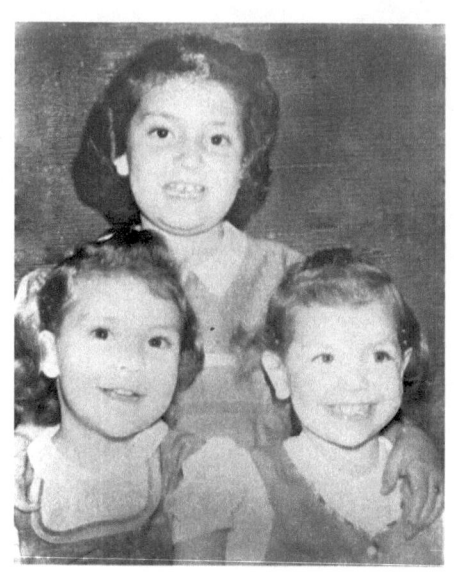

Photo of (left to right) me, Anne, and Betty, 1955

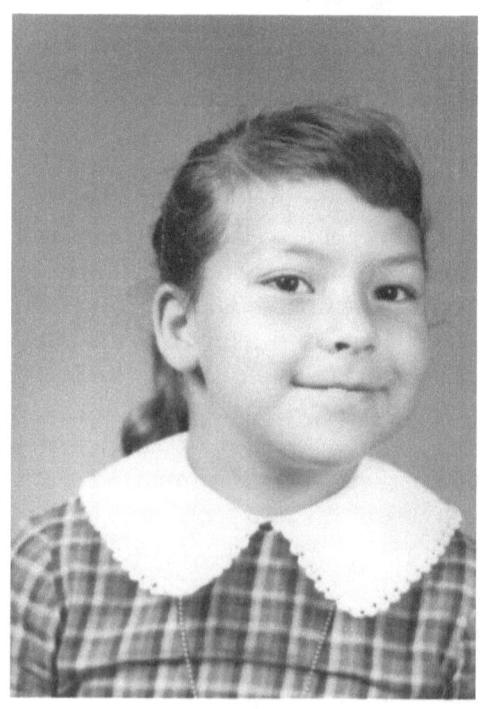

Me, 1958

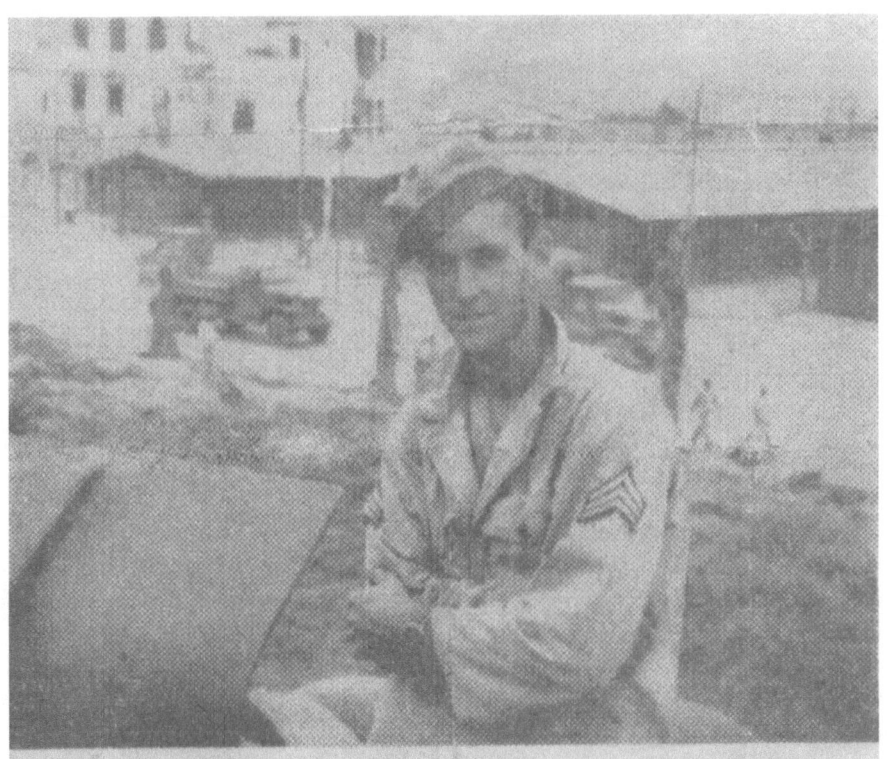

Serving in Philippines

From worker in a TNT plant to gun commander, Sgt. James H. Burton, so nof Mrs. Oscar Burton, route 2, Karnack, serves in the Philippines as part of an automatic Weapons battalion in Maj. Gen. William F. Marquat's 14th anti-aircraft command. In the background are the ruins of Manila. (14th AA Photo)

Photo)

My father's photo when he was serving in
the Army in the Philippines, 1944

CHAPTER 3

Living With Big Momma And Little Daddy (Age 10-12)

Living with my grandparents was quite an adjustment since I really didn't know them very well. We had never gone to spend the summer with them, I didn't remember getting any birthday or Christmas presents from them, so who were they? All of us arrived in Elysian Fields, Texas, at my grandparents' house late in the evening in mom's almost new white 1959 Chevy Impala. After the car was unloaded, she told us bye and we were hustled to bed by Big Momma. Mom went back to Marshall and we didn't see her for over three years. Big Momma took us to visit her in the hospital in Shreveport, La., after she tried to overdose on sleeping pills. Big Momma told us she had a nervous breakdown. Is there really such a thing as a nervous breakdown?

I was in the fifth grade and Anne had just started high school. My grandparents doted over Anne I guess because she was older. During our stay she was the apple of their eye. Betty and I were treated like orphans and I always felt like I was unwanted and a burden on them. It wasn't really Anne's fault but when you're a little kid it just doesn't seem fair.

Little Daddy and Big Momma owned a five acre farm. Two acres they plowed for the vegetable garden, about two acres were for the farm animals, and the three bedroom, one bath home with a torn up garage which served as a chicken coop sit on the rest of it. There was also an old outhouse which only Little Daddy used. I didn't know what an outhouse was until then. This was the early '60's and no one used outhouses anymore, or so I thought. Much to my surprise there was no running water in the bathroom. There was a sink, a tub, and a toilet with pipes, but none of the plumbing was connected to the well. The kitchen had running water, but not the bathroom. Apparently, my grandparents thought connecting the bathroom to the well would draw too much water out and run it dry. We could take a bath but we had to haul water into the bathroom from the kitchen sink. Grandmother made Betty and I bathe together. We could use the toilet but once again, we had to bring water from the kitchen to flush. And forget about using the bathroom sink, it wasn't worth the effort. We brushed our teeth in the kitchen sink. Getting dressed for school was quite a chore with the three of us fighting over the meager facilities. Little Daddy usually resorted to the outhouse instead of fighting for time in the bathroom. At night, he would take his pistol with him in case there were snakes or wild animals.

My grandparents were in their early 30's with three children during the Great Depression of 1929, so because of that experience they didn't spend a dime unless it was absolutely necessary. They believed in paying as you go and being self sufficient. I remember the first few times we went to the grocery store with Big Momma. She bought less than ten items: flour, sugar, toilet paper, laundry soap, coffee, bananas, dish soap, snuff, and Little Daddy's tobacco. Everything else we either grew or raised on the farm. I also have to mention Little Daddy owned and operated a filling station in Bethany, Louisiana, which is just a few miles from Elysian Fields but in a different state. For those of you who don't know what a filling station is, it's a gas station with an attendant who checked your oil, pumped your gas, and washed your windshield. Something unheard of today. Once or twice a month, Betty and I would help Little Daddy at the filling station and get a candy bar and red pop for our pay. We loved running the manual cash register and listening to the bells ring when you opened it. Little Daddy believed in the barter system. He would accept farm animals or farm equipment for payment. Since Bethany is a small city and he knew everybody in town he would accept trade in lieu of cash or occasionally, allow credit. Little Daddy usually broke even or came out slightly ahead every month. After all, it was the only filling station in town.

Sundays were devoted to religion. Little Daddy didn't go to church but Big Momma sang in the choir at the Baptist church and was there every time the doors were open. In other words, Sundays were a day of worship and everybody (except Little Daddy) attended church; Sunday morning, Sunday evening, and Wednesday evening. Until now, I had never set foot in a church. This was all new to me but I was baptized when I was twelve years old in Big Momma's Baptist church.

I guess I should describe my grandparents. They were Scottish Irish mix and their parents migrated to the United States in the mid 1800's. Big Momma was about 5'5", brown hair and eyes, wore glasses and orthopedic shoes, weighed about 250 pounds, walked like Chester on "Gunsmoke", and dipped snuff. She was a strong willed, hard working, Christian woman. She was also a strong disciplinarian and had a quick right hand which she used to slap Betty and me in the face a few times for talking back to her. Little Daddy was about 5'9", brown hair, green eyes, also wore glasses, weighed approximately 150 pounds, and smoked. He only had one eye; his left eye was sewn shut after he injured it as a child on a barb wire fence. He smoked and rolled his own cigarettes from Prince Albert tobacco. I always thought the two made a very odd couple. I suspect Big Momma walked like Chester because she had arthritis but neither of them ever went to the doctor. I also suspect she was a diabetic because she always drank Dr. Pepper, ate Payday candy bars, and complained about her sugar but at ten years old I had no idea what she was talking about. They had four children, all girls, however one (Ruth) died at the age of six from diphtheria. Big Momma talked about her frequently—how hard it was to just sit and watch her die because there was no cure or vaccination at the time. I'm guessing that in 1961, Big Momma and Little Daddy were in their late fifties or early sixties, but seemed a lot older. One thing I noticed right away, Little Daddy slept on a cot in the living room and Big Momma slept on a full bed in what was meant to be the dinning room. The three bedrooms had furniture in them but looked like they were never used. The bedroom near the screened in back porch had an old bed in it but the room was primarily used as a junk room. Since central heat and air conditioning really didn't exist yet, every room had a small gas heater and there were several fans strategically placed around the house that we used in the summer.

Big Momma used to get dressed in her bedroom (the dinning room) every morning and wasn't modest. She wore slips with no bra, huge underwear with no elastic in the legs, and always a dress, either her work dresses or her Sunday best. She never wore pants and Anne wasn't allowed to either. Betty and I were allowed to wear shorts and pants but I guess at a certain age it was no longer acceptable. Watching Big Momma get dressed for church was a sight to see. It was always the same—blue or black dress with matching shoes and purse, some type of Jackie Kennedy hat, rouge, red lipstick, clip on earrings, false teeth out of the jar, knee high nylons and a string of white pearls around her neck. I don't know where she got those pearls, but they meant the world to her. Whenever she got dressed up, those pearls were always around her neck.

Sundays were a day of rest, so after church we all came home and had a very large fantastic lunch. Lunch usually consisted of fried chicken (the chicken we had killed and cleaned the day before), mashed potatoes or potato salad, fresh beans or peas, corn bread, cobbler or pie, watermelon, and iced tea. After lunch was nap time for a couple of hours, then it was time to get ready to go back to church. With all that food and a nap no wonder I was chunky. Actually, I got fat because I wasn't use to all that food. Big Momma started calling me "lard ass" after a couple of months which was really hurtful. We wore the same clothes to evening services that we wore to morning services in order to cut down on the laundry. If you got your clothes dirty during morning services or forgot to hang them up when you got home, too bad, that's the way you went to evening services.

Living with my grandparents was all about work, something I wasn't used to. I didn't realize how much work could be squeezed into 15-16 hours. Saturdays were the worse because that was laundry and house cleaning day on top of everything else. Doing the laundry was horrible since Big Momma had a wringer washer out on the screened back porch and no dryer. So, we washed the clothes in the washer, then took them all outside to two large wash tubs filled with water and bluing to rinse them, and then hung them out on the clothes lines. There were only two clothes lines and a ton of clothes now that the three of us had moved in. Since there wasn't enough clothes line, about half of the clothes had to be hung on the bushes in the back yard. Only problem with that was if we didn't get the clothes in after two or three hours, the chickens would fly up on the bushes and poop on the clean clothes. Doing laundry was horrible. I don't know why Little Daddy didn't buy a dryer or at least add more clothes lines. After laundry came house cleaning which took another couple of hours. This wasn't cleaning like you think of today. The old farm house was a dust bowl so the primary cleaning tools were a dust rag, a dust mop, and a broom. The broom was for the area rugs since she didn't have a vacuum cleaner. Oh, by the way, the laundry and house cleaning took place after the eggs were gathered, the chickens were fed, the cows were milked and fed, and the pigs were slopped. The vegetable garden was normally only worked through the week.

Anne was usually out with her friends on Friday and Saturday nights. Since she was in high school she had more freedom. That was great for her but Betty and I had no friends and went nowhere. Saturday evening for us was watching TV with the grandparents until around eight at night then getting a bath and going to bed. After our bath, the water was generally like mud particularly in the summer since we were outside all day. The summers in East Texas and Louisiana are hot and humid, so the dirt stuck to us in little balls around our necks and in our arm pits. We were always filthy from working on the farm, climbing trees, or riding the oil wells on my grandparents' property.

This is hard to say but during the three plus years I lived with Little Daddy and Big Momma, I don't remember any visits or phone calls from either of my parents and no affection from my grandparents. There were no praises, no hugs, no kisses, no gifts, no birthday parties, no Christmas tree, no new clothes except a few things needed for school, no nothing. The first Christmas there Betty and I asked Big Momma about our Christmas presents and she handed us an old Sears and Roebuck catalogue, a pair of kids' scissors, and some Elmer's glue and told us to go sit on the living room floor and cut paper dolls. Actually, that

---

19

turned out to be a great Christmas present. We played with those paper dolls for months. Of course there were no allowances either. Things I remember I liked: watermelon and homemade ice cream parties in the summer, hula hoop, Louisiana coffee brewing on the stove, and clean, white heated sheets.

When I was twelve years old, I started my period. No one had ever told me anything about sex or what a menstrual cycle was, so of course when I saw blood in my underwear I was horrified. I told Anne who sort of explained it and gave me a couple of her Kotex. When those Kotex were gone, Big Momma refused to buy me anymore. Instead, she tore an old sheet in strips and told me to fold one of the strips in quarters and pin it in my underwear. At night, all the used strips were soaked in bleach and washed and I wore them again. This continued a couple of months until she finally broke down and bought me a box of Kotex. During the time that I was on my period and had to wear the strips of sheet, I smelled like dead meat. At school it was difficult to change my strips of sheet so I would try not to get out of my seat and I always sat with my legs crossed where nobody would smell me. That was disgusting. Big Momma did not spend a dime she didn't have to spend. Being a survivor of the Great Depression had made its mark on her. I understand that today, but not when I was living with her.

About this same time, I asked Big Momma to teach me to drive. She had a fairly new tan Comet with a column shift. A column shift was the forerunner of a stick shift which of course has a clutch. She let me drive to and from the filling station which was about two miles down the road and eventually I got the hang of the clutch. In addition to feeling grown up by driving, it got me out of the back seat. I mentioned earlier that Big Momma dipped snuff and since she didn't have a spit can in the car, she would roll the driver's window down and spit out. Betty and I always rode in the back seat with our windows down in the summer and we got sprayed with her spit out snuff. Now Betty was in the back seat by herself and could move to the other side of the car to avoid the spit.

The only television was black and white and was in the living room where Little Daddy slept. Therefore, he controlled the television and what was watched. When he came home from the filling station for lunch he would time it where he was through eating and ready to watch "Let's Make A Deal" with Monte Hall then the local news. In the evening, all of us piled in the living room to watch "What's My Line", "I Love Lucy", "Red Skelton", and a few others. Betty and I took our pillows and would lie on the floor in front of the set. One night programming was interrupted and President John Kennedy came on the air. While writing this novel, I decided to describe a few major historical events which occurred during my lifetime and denote them as Historical Markers. So, here is the first. Historical Marker #1: The Cuban Missile Crisis, 1962. During his television broadcast, President Kennedy warned the nation of a possible nuclear attack from Russia and Cuba and said we should be prepared to go to the bomb shelters. He advised us to stock the shelters with enough canned food and water to last at least three months. President Kennedy even told us how the shelter should be constructed in order to withstand a nuclear bomb—out of bricks or thick cement. I was scared to death even though I had no idea what a nuclear bomb was. After hearing President Kennedy's broadcast, we stocked our storm shelter, which was definitely not a bomb shelter, and hoped for the best. I am certainly glad that catastrophe was avoided.

Big Momma died in 1974, while I was in Guam from complications resulting from a fall down the back porch steps. Little Daddy died about ten years later from cancer. I believe I was in Washington, D.C. when he died and found out after the fact. Consequently, I did not attend either funeral. I heard that when Little Daddy died, their three daughters descended on that little farm house like a pack of vultures and picked it to the bone. Mom and her two sisters (both were quite wealthy) fought over what little was left behind by their parents. I think the three of them agreed to sell the property for little of nothing and divide the money. I am glad I wasn't around to witness their behavior.

Historical Marker #2: November 22, 1963, President John F. Kennedy was assassinated in Dallas, Texas. I was in the sixth grade. After lunch, our teacher turned on the television and Walter Cronkite was announcing the horrific news that President Kennedy had been shot and had died at around 1:00 pm Texas time.

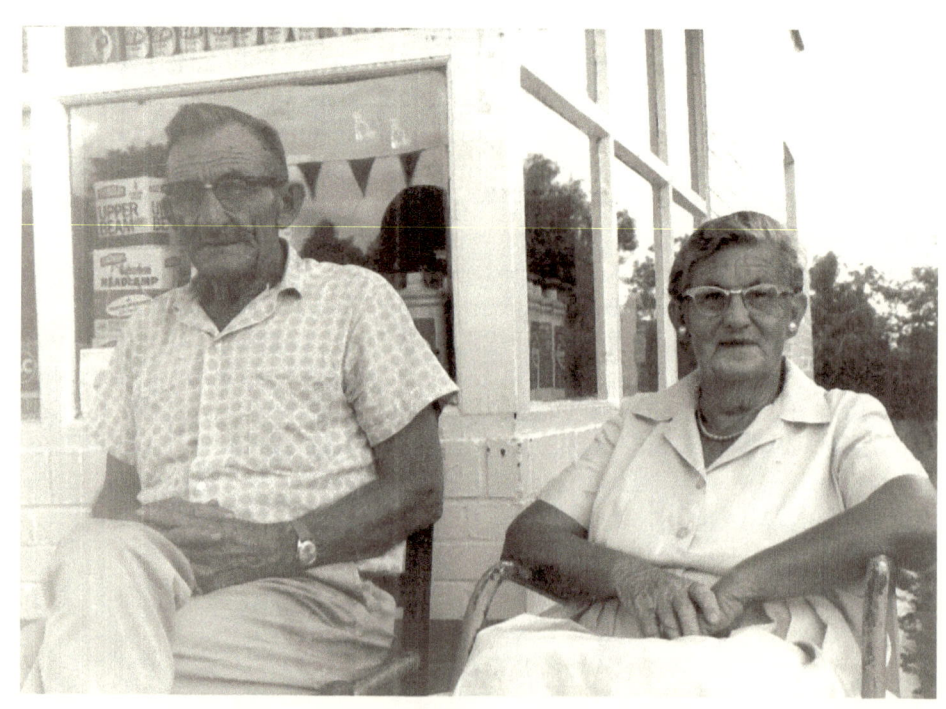

Big Momma and Little Daddy, 1962

CHAPTER 4

The Really Terrible Teens (Age 13-17)

The last summer I was at my grandparents all three of us were sent to my great aunt and uncle's house about 50 miles away to help them in the cotton fields. They owned several acres of land, part of it was a cotton field and the other was the typical farm like my grandparents. Uncle Randy and Aunt Alma were their names. Their primary source of income was from the cotton and they owned their own gin. Anne, Betty and I had been there about three weeks when out of the blue Little Daddy came to pick us up and take us back to Elysian Fields. Quite frankly, I was more than ready to leave because working in the cotton fields was definitely hard work. Anne told me recently that the reason Little Daddy came to pick us up was because she had been sexually molested by Uncle Randy. I thought Uncle Randy and Aunt Alma were hard working, decent, Christian people but apparently I was wrong. Uncle Randy was in his 60's and just an old pervert. I guess perverts come in all ages, races, and socio-economic levels. I never saw or heard anything about Uncle Randy or Aunt Alma again or remember being told they had passed.

About two weeks later, mother appeared out of nowhere and took Betty and I back to Marshall and the house on Fannin Street. Anne chose to stay with my grandparents and graduate high school at Elysian Fields. Looking back, I think my grandparents were tired of taking care of the three of us and told mother to come get Betty and I. School was about to start and I was growing up. I would be starting the eighth grade—Junior High School!

I don't remember much about the eighth grade other than I was overweight starting a new school with wore out clothes, and having only one friend, Marsha, a neighbor. Since Anne had stayed in Elysian Fields with my grandparents and mom was either working or out on a date, Betty and I were pretty much on our own. We rode our bicycles until dark or played with our Barbie dolls with

Marsha. If we needed anything, our great aunt Ollie lived about a block away. Betty and I would go over there for something to eat in the evening then go home and get ready for bed. That year I really don't remember seeing much of mom. I guess she had gotten used to not having us around. When mom was home, she always seemed to be mad about something. I remember getting many spankings with the belt or a switch off one of the trees in the yard. I guess life just wasn't being good to her.

At the end of the school year, Anne had who graduated from high school that year, announced she wanted to go to nursing school in Tyler, Texas. She had received a scholarship to a three year RN program and would reside on campus. At the end of the summer, we sold most of our furniture, gave the house back to the bank, packed up the car and moved to Tyler. We found a partially furnished apartment and mom got a job at Kentucky Fried Chicken. She brought home leftovers almost every night from KFC for Betty and me to eat for dinner and after a few months I couldn't stand the site of that chicken. When school started I went to high school but Betty was still in junior high. This was the first time that we had been separated and it was a long, lonely year. Mom had a couple of boyfriends that year and one or two actually moved into the apartment for awhile. They were all drunks she had met at bars. Betty and I didn't like them and they certainly didn't like us. We didn't see much of Anne anymore. She only came home for an occasional Sunday visit, so it was Betty and I taking care of the drunks while mom was at work. One of them, Neal, went on a drunken binge and stayed on our sofa for at least two weeks drinking, smoking, vomiting, cussing, and wetting his pants. Neal and his older brother owned a flower shop and nursery in Tyler. He would have been a millionaire if he wasn't a drunk. Neal was disgusting but mom just kept telling us how rich he was and how rich we would be when they got married. Well, she did marry him not long after that and we all packed up again and moved into an old house he had recently purchased. This was the first of six stepfathers or as I started calling them "frogs". This one burned the house down for the insurance money the following year and went to prison. Betty and I had to testify against him in court since we saw him with the three gasoline cans he used to start the fire. Mother didn't get a dime from him. You would think she would learn, but she never did. Mom kept looking for men to support her where she wouldn't have to work. I don't know why she thought like that, but she told Betty and I many times she would eventually find a rich man to marry and we would all "live high on the hog". It never happened. During my high school years, we packed up and moved about every six or seven months, enduring one stepfather after another. The only possessions we had were a few dishes, linens, towels, and our clothes. I remember one time mom came home and told us to we had to move right then and to throw all our clothes into the middle of the bed, tie the sheets around all of it and throw it out the bedroom window. We lived in a two story apartment at that time. Mom would stand underneath the bedroom window, grab the tied up sheets and throw them in the trunk or back seat of the car. She then went into the apartment packed the dishes in the kitchen and we were out of there in a little over an hour. I'm guessing she hadn't paid the rent in several months. Another time when we were living with one of my stepfathers by the name of Dick, mom packed our clothes in trash bags and loaded her car late at night when Dick was asleep. After loading the car, she quietly woke Betty and me up and hurried us out to the car and started driving off. Then, out of nowhere I hear a couple of loud pops and look back to see Dick standing in the middle of the driveway shooting at the car. Thank goodness he was a lousy marksman and missed. I'm going to take a wild guess and say she took the money out of his wallet is why he was shooting at us. Dick was wealthy and always kept about a thousand dollars in his wallet. He liked to pull it out and show it to us. She had probably been stealing from him for months. Mom was working as a receptionist at a doctor's office at the time and had the keys to the front door, so that is where we spent the night. The three of us slept on the examining beds at the doctor's office. We were gypsies and thieves. Mom kept thinking if she kissed the right frog he would turn into a prince and we would all be rich. Unfortunately, life doesn't work that way. With each move, Betty and I changed schools. To say the least, my junior high and high school years were chaotic.

After a couple of semesters, Anne dropped out of her RN program because her grades slipped below the required 3.0. She moved outside Tyler, changed colleges and became a licensed medical lab technician instead. Anne did eventually complete her four year degree later in life. Soon after changing colleges she married her first husband, Victor who was drafted into the Army not long after they married. Victor decided to join the Air Force in lieu of the Army and shipped out to Thailand a few months later. About the same time Victor left for Thailand, Anne told us she was pregnant. While Victor was in Thailand, Anne lived with his aunt and uncle in Jacksonville, about 25 miles outside of Tyler. During this period, their son Paul was born. After Victor returned from Thailand, the Air Force transferred him to Dover, Delaware and Anne, Paul, and Victor spent the next two or three years up north. Unfortunately, their marriage ended and Anne and Paul returned to Tyler at the end of Victor's tour in Delaware. The year was 1966 and the Viet Nam War was getting hot and heavy but it wasn't yet affecting me. Anne never came back home so Betty and I were left to our vices; smoking, drinking, skipping school, staying out most of the night, etc.

When I was 16, I took driver's education in high school and mom helped me buy my first car. It was a navy blue, 1967, Ford Mustang. What a car! Mom made the down payment with the understanding I make the monthly car payments. In order to do that, I needed a job. At the time, she was working at El Chico Restaurant in Tyler. You got it—mom got Betty and me a job at the restaurant as part-time waitresses. If you've ever worked as a waitress, you know that the meat of your salary is your tips. Since we were young and cute (I had lost about 20 pounds), we made a killing. The other female waitresses were in their 40's and 50's and not much to look at. Since we were working, it relieved mom from having to give us money for anything. In other words, Betty and I were working and supporting ourselves from this point on.

Having a car, a part-time job, and no parental supervision was a recipe for disaster. Betty and I quickly turned into juvenile delinquents. We started smoking, drinking, skipping school, hanging out with college students, and we rarely came home. In 1967, the legal age to buy alcoholic beverages was 18. We were never carded and were always able to purchase anything we wanted. Under the dash of the Mustang was a black box which held two fifths and a couple cans of Coke or four cans of beer. I don't know what this black box was intended to be used for but it became our liquor hiding place. The police pulled us over a couple of times, searched the car and never looked in the black box. Once we got pulled over for speeding and of course both of us were drinking a mixed drink. While the cop was running the plates, Betty and I came up with a plan. While the policeman was on my side of the car asking for my driver's license, Betty would quietly poor the drinks out her window. This plan actually worked. In the late '60's, cops in small towns were quite tolerant of wild teens and would usually just tell you to get home. And that was what he did. I didn't get a ticket for speeding and he never noticed the mixed drinks Betty had poured out her window; or at least I don't think he did.

Good thing I am intelligent. I was a sophomore in high school taking college prep classes, making As and Bs and skipping school at least one day a week. When I got caught, I would opt for the three licks instead of the five day suspension. This was back in the day when corporal punishment was allowed. I opted for the licks in order to prevent the school from attempting to contact mom. Besides, the licks with a wooden paddle didn't hurt that much and my grades didn't suffer. I was more concerned about my grades than them contacting mom which was virtually impossible anyway because she was seldom home, we didn't have a home phone, and I intercepted the mail. When I skipped school, I would get the assignments from one of the other students and turn the work in late. In order to obtain the missed assignments, I was required to do that person's homework as well. I helped Betty with her assignments too since she was usually with me when I skipped school. This is the way I made it through high school.

As long as Betty and I brought home good report cards and kept working, which we did, we could do just about anything we wanted. That was all that was expected of us. Mom was too busy looking for her Prince Charming but always coming up with the ugly ass frog. The only time she found out Betty and I had skipped school was when we went skinny dipping in the lake near the school and the vice principal drove by and saw us. There were about ten kids with a cooler filled with beer sitting on the side of the small lake near the school. He must have had a stroke when he saw that many students out of school half naked, with beer and cigarettes, the car radios blasting, and all of us buzzed and dancing around. I remember he stopped his car for a couple of minutes and looked right at me. When I went back to school the next day, I was immediately called to the principal's office and handed a five day suspension. There was very little conversation and no option for licks. That was the end of my junior year. I made sure I was never caught skipping school again. Needless to say, there was no way to hide this from mom since my grades would take a hit. When I told her, she hit the roof and took the keys to the Mustang away from me for a week. Fortunately, after begging my teachers, I was able to make up most of the class work and my grades only dropped one letter.

At the beginning of my senior year, mom changed jobs and met another one of her frogs so we moved again. This time it was to Whitehouse, a small city about eight miles outside of Tyler. The high school only had 350 students. Needless to say, Betty and I didn't like it so we made frequent trips to Tyler to hang out with our friends and cruise Main Street. Whitehouse was very boring. We were still working at El Chico's on the weekend so we usually stayed over at one of our friends' house on Saturday night. Betty and I were thick as thieves and bad to the bone. By this time, mom had lost all control over us and didn't really care where we were or what we were doing. I guess her and her new boyfriend were thankful for the peace and quite.

My senior year was awesome. Betty and I dressed in hot mini skirts, wore lots of makeup, and stayed out most of the night—usually with college students. Betty even managed to land a couple of dates with one of the cute local police officers. Needless to say we never got pulled over again unless it was him wanting to talk to Betty. Since we were working and splitting the car expenses, both of us had plenty of money. El Chico's was fun now. Betty and I would make fun of the Mexican cooks' English which prompted them to throw dinner rolls at us and a food fight ensued. Almost every Friday night there was a food fight in the kitchen. The manager of the restaurant at that time was a really cute Hispanic named Gilbert. Gilbert was in his late twenties and married but he always flirted with Betty and me. He also never said a word about the food fights except telling us to clean it up. Gilbert was cool.

When we weren't raising havoc at El Chico's, Betty and I were preying on the unsuspecting public. When we ran out of money and were hungry, we would steal food. We had three sure fire ways to eat and not pay. Our favorite place was the local Piggly Wiggly grocery store after ten at night. Around that time most of the shoppers had left and there were only a few store employees in the store. It was amazing how much food we could consume in less than five minutes. We would grab a package of lunch meat and cheese then head over to the produce department to graze. Our plan, if we got caught was for me to fake an epileptic seizure as a diversion. I actually had to do that one time. The manager of the grocery store caught Betty and I chowing down on the grapes and insisted we pay for them or he was calling the police. So I started rolling my eyes to the back of my head, fell to the floor and started flopping around, while Betty screamed that I was having another seizure. It worked like a charm. Betty pretended to put one of my pills under my tongue to stop the seizure and the manager apologized while he escorted us to our car. After all that excitement, he had forgotten about all the food we had eaten.

The next best way to steal food was to go into a nice restaurant and look for an old couple to sit next to. Once we spotted our target, we would sit down, order a large meal, and tell the waitress/waiter that our grandparents were buying us dinner and to give them the check. We would point them out to the wait person and wave at the old couple to make it look legit, then eat hurriedly and leave before the old couple had finished their meal and got the check. This always worked. Older people don't want to cause trouble and they rarely remember what a couple of kids who waved at them looked like.

As a last resort, Betty and I would go to the Sonic and listen for order numbers and when the person or couple who ordered the food was distracted, pretend to be their kids, pick up their food and leave quickly. Of course, the clerk would stand there for a couple of minutes waiting on the real customer to come pay for the food, hence giving Betty and I time to make it to the car and drive off without the headlights. No point going to all this trouble if the clerk could see your tag number. This tactic was risky but we never got caught.

As I look back, it amazes me that we were able to get away with so much. Stealing food soon became a game which we tired of. The rush was gone so we moved up to bigger thrills. Betty and I decided it would be fun to ride the railroad tracks in the Mustang. One night we stopped and got two fifths of Jim Beam and one coke and asked a couple of guys we knew if they wanted to go cruising. Of course the fools agreed, particularly when they found out we had plenty of Beam. The Supremes and the Beatles were blaring on the car radio and after a few drinks Betty and I asked the guys if they were man enough for a ride on the railroad. No seventeen year old boy is going to say no. We talked them into letting a little air out of the tires so the car would stay on the tracks and took off for the ride of our lives. I let one of the guys drive and was sitting in the back seat. He drove the car up to a railroad crossing and jumped on the tracks. The width of the Mustang was a perfect fit on the tracks. The four of us rode the tracks about ten or twelve miles but decided not to continue to press our luck and jumped off the tracks at the next crossing. Looking back, that was a really stupid thing to do but a real rush not knowing if we were going to run into a train on the track and if we did what we would do. I might as well have been playing Russian roulette. Rush or no rush, I never did that again. After I sobered up I realized how dangerous it was. Instead, I started drag racing the Mustang in the illegal Saturday night races on Main Street in Tyler. I seldom won but that Mustang was one hot mama. This was a real high and I was completely sober. When you're 17, life is a bowl of cherries and you believe you are completely invincible. Also, this was during the height of the Viet Nam War and the mind set of the youth at that time was live today because you might die tomorrow—the beliefs of a true baby boomer.

Historical Markers 3 and 4: In 1968, Dr. Martin Luther King Jr. and Robert Kennedy were assassinated; one in Memphis and one in Los Angeles. This was a loss of two great men—one a well known civil rights leader and the other a presidential candidate. In 1987, while working with the Memphis Police Department, I had the opportunity to see the Loraine Hotel where Dr. King was assassinated. The second floor where Dr. King was shot always has a fresh wreath of flowers in front of the room where he died.

In February of 1969, mother decided she had had enough of the two wild kids. I really don't know what brought this on except she was single again and was noticing Betty and I were seldom home. Mom told me that since I would soon be eighteen, I needed to decide what I was going to do with myself after graduation. She made it clear I wasn't staying at home and there certainly wasn't any money for college. Mom gave me the option of the street, juvenile custody, or the military. I chose the military. The U.S. Air Force to be exact. I took the entrance exam that month, passed it, and entered the delayed entry program in February, 1969. To get into the Air Force, I had to be 18, a high school graduate, and ten pounds lighter. My grades were still As and Bs and once I quit drinking like a fish, I quickly lost the ten pounds. In 1969, less than one percent of the military was female. The thought of being one of a few, wearing a uniform, traveling, and having a steady income was very appealing to me. I shipped out to boot camp in San Antonio, Texas, on May 22, 1969. My high school diploma was mailed to mom since I left before the graduation ceremony.

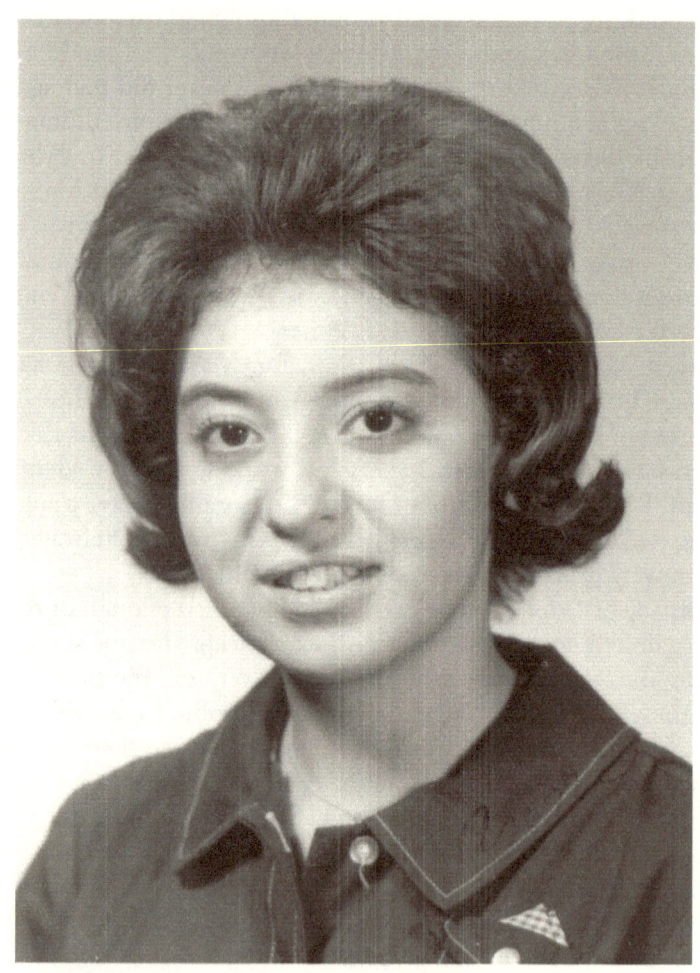

Anne, 1964

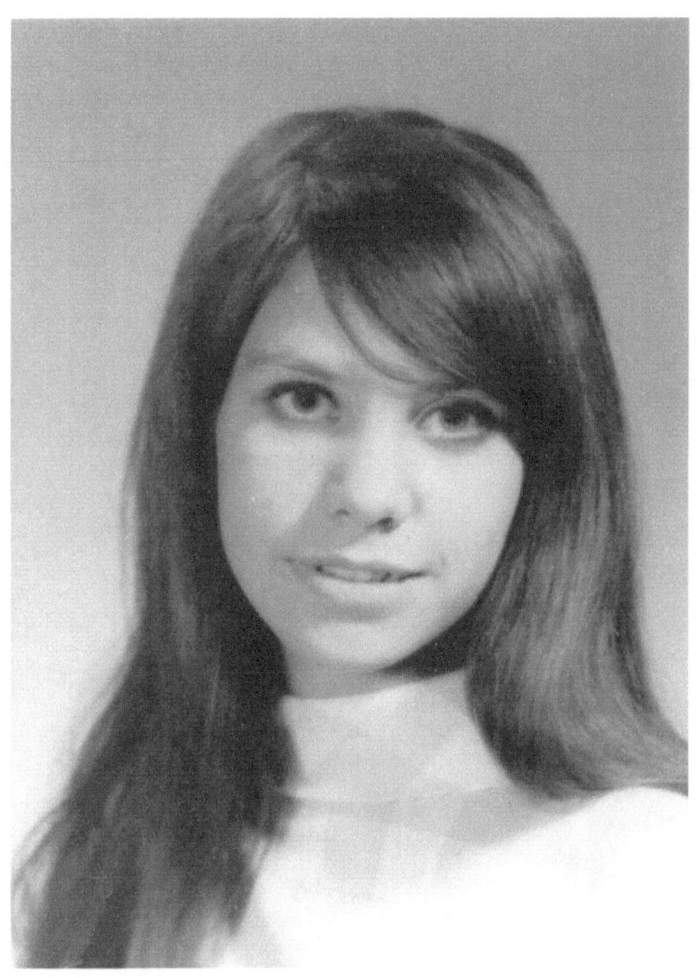

Betty, 1968

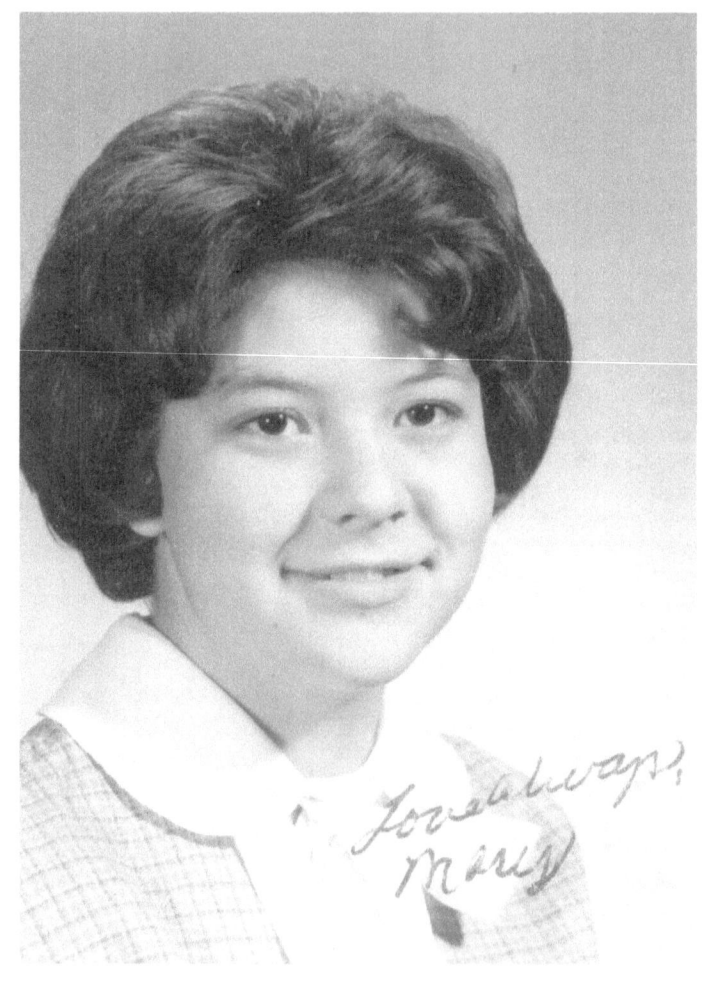

Me, 1968

CHAPTER 5

Wild Thing Joins the Air Force
(Age 18-22)

I shipped out from the Dallas Greyhound Bus Station that afternoon and arrived at Lackland Air Force Base, San Antonio, Texas the next morning around three. I had just spent all night on a bus full of men with only one stop and no food or water. Including myself, there were only three women on that bus and over 30 men. I was tired and hungry but no one cared. I told one of the drill instructors that I needed to use the bathroom and was hungry. He promptly told me to shut my "fucking" mouth and keep it shut unless I was spoken to and anytime I talked to a drill instructor I needed to begin and end responses with a "mam" or "sir".

The Air Force was part of the Army until 1964, and was called the Army Air Corp. In 1969, most of the drill instructors (D.I.s) were carried over from the Army and mean as a junk yard dog. After debarking the bus, a female D.I. took charge of me and the other women. I noticed right away that the female D.I.s looked a lot like the male D.I.s with one exception—they all wore bright red lipstick. They didn't have on any other makeup, just that awful bright red lipstick. I thought this was very odd. We were lined up and marched to the female barracks, thrown a sandwich, a half pint of milk and some sheets. We all had ten minutes to eat, get the sheets on the bed, get undressed and get into bed. I got about two hours sleep that night because at five a.m. a couple of the female D.I.s threw metal trash cans into our rooms to wake us up. They were kicking the trash cans, blowing whistles, and yelling "get up recruits". Well, this was not exactly what the recruiter had told me boot camp was going to be like and I didn't care for it one little bit.

The new recruits were called "newbies". That morning, after the horrific wake up call, we were marched outside in formation for revelry, then to breakfast, then to get uniforms, then to lunch, etc. Finally, around 5:15 in the evening, our class was put back into formation for retreat and the day was finally coming to a close. "Lights Out" was at 9 p.m. sharp. This meant in your bed with the lights out and asleep. Boot Camp was six long weeks in the summer in south Texas in 90 to 100 degree heat. Part of our training was learning how to march. We marched on a huge cement parking lot in that heat for hour upon hours. Some of the girls passed out, others threw up. It didn't matter, the training continued. Learning how to march in formation is not easy. The first thing you have to learn is not to walk on the balls of your feet. Your heels have to hit the ground first so you don't pop up and down. The D.I.s were constantly yelling "heel, toe, heel, toe". Then you have to remember to always start out on your left foot, look straight ahead and swing your arms. This takes a lot of practice which is why we were on the drill pad in the Texas heat at least six hours a day. We were given salt tablets and jungle hats in lieu of water, rest or shade. This was during Viet Nam and drill instructors were permitted to train new recruits pretty much any way they saw fit. The D.I.s told us from day one that they were our momma and papa and the Air Force was our new family. This was part of the resocialization process. About thirty percent of our class dropped out. I really thought about it but I didn't want to go back to my old life in Tyler. The six weeks past quickly and I only got in trouble a couple of times for refusing to wear the hooker red lipstick and not remembering "heel first". One of the drill instructors made me stand at attention while she put that hooker red lipstick on my lips. I looked like a clown. For refusing to wear the red lipstick, she instructed me to clean the bathroom with a tooth brush and powder cleaner that night after dinner. I didn't get through cleaning that bathroom until around one in the morning and had to get up at five. I didn't care, that lipstick on an eighteen year old was tacky and I refused to wear it. The day for orders for "A" school arrived and I was so excited. This school was the training for your career in the Air Force. The one thing I had told the recruiter I didn't want was food service. I should have known. My orders were for "Cook" with a school in Ft. Lee, Virginia. I was really ticked off. Being a cook was insulting. It was the lowest level of training reserved for dummies. I was smarter than this. So I went to Ft. Lee with an attitude. Cook school was eight weeks then my permanent duty station was McGuire Air Force Base, New Jersey.

In the summer of 1969, the war in Viet Nam was going badly. Hundreds of brave young men were being sent home in body bags and wooden boxes every month. The sentiment regarding the war was changing. There were protesters popping up everywhere in the U.S. and the public started despising anyone wearing a military uniform. I was oblivious to all of this. Since this was my first time away from home and out of the state of Texas, I was having too good a time to think about the war.

Ft. Lee is located outside Richmond, Va., and it was hot and muggy when I arrived the middle of July. Of course there was no air conditioning in the old World War II barracks in which we were housed, not even window units. In 1969, central air wasn't the norm but window units existed. Every room had two windows and a fan so we sweated a lot. I quickly made friends with one of my roommates, Libby. She was in her mid twenties, divorced, and Army. Libby had dyed black hair, wore way too much make up, was very sexy, and loved men. I don't know why but I was instantly attracted to Libby. She seemed like a whole lot of fun.

We were out of boot camp and had a little more freedom but not much. All of the troops were expected to be at revelry at 5 a.m., retreat at 5:30 p.m., and in bed for bed check at 9 p.m. These hours didn't allow much time for having fun, so Libby and I decided to make our own hours. We decided that nine o'clock at night was way too early for bed. Libby had a couple of wigs and wig heads which were perfect to put in our beds along with a couple of extra pillows to make it look like we were in bed asleep. We started keeping an overnight bag packed and ready. Libby and I would go to the base softball games and meet lots of really cute, sexy men. We were only interested in the ones who had cars and apartments off base. After the game, we would arrange for them to pick us up near the barracks at 8:45. So, around 9:00 p.m., while the duty personnel were busy doing bed check, Libby and I would grab our overnight bags and slip out the bathroom window for a night of fun. In 1969, HIV/AIDS didn't exist so safe sex meant taking your birth control pills. Condoms which had been in use for centuries didn't exist for us either. This was the period of "Free Love" and no one used condoms. The word condom is Latin meaning receptacle and mass production of condoms began in 1844. But of course my ignorant butt had never heard of or seen a condom. At this time, I was a virgin, had my birth control pills, and was dying to get laid. Libby was always horny and men just seemed to migrate toward her. Under these circumstances, picking up men was a snap. What red blooded young man wouldn't be attracted to two hot, willing, sexy, young sluts? I lost my virginity that month to an Army sergeant whose name I can't remember and who I never saw or heard from again. He was shipping out to Viet Nam and I gave him my high school graduation ring and promised to write. I always wondered what happened to him and if he made it back from the war. Stuffing our beds and climbing out the bathroom window worked like a charm for three or four weeks. That is until Libby and I came back to the barracks around two in the morning drunk as a skunk. For the life of us we couldn't get through that small bathroom window which was about three feet off the ground. So we dropped our overnight bags on the floor and the two of us

—

fell in after them laughing like crazy. Everything was funny right then. Needless to say all that racket woke up the duty person as well as half the barracks. The female duty officer helped us up off the bathroom floor then promptly notified the officer in charge of our barracks what had happened. The girl on duty didn't even know we were out of the barracks because she was fooled by the wig and stuffed bed. I wish I had of taken a picture of her face when she escorted us back to our room, turned on the light, and pulled back the covers. She was really ticked. Libby and I were so drunk all of this was extremely funny. We were on the floor rolling around laughing. We were so wasted we couldn't walk and had to crawl to our room. The girl on duty relayed to us that the commanding officer would be dealing with this incident the next morning.

The next morning came way too soon. Since Libby and I didn't get to bed until after two in the morning, five o'clock seemed like just ten minutes sleep. The nights we came in late Libby and I didn't bother to put our complete uniform on for revelry, just our boots, hat, and raincoat. We had been doing this for a good three weeks, so this morning was no different. The two of us went down to formation half dressed like always which proved to be a huge mistake. After revelry, the commanding officer asked Libby and I to open our raincoats for a uniform inspection. She must have known that we were still in our tee shirts and underwear which is what we slept in every night. Libby and I reluctantly opened our raincoats and waited for the feathers to fly. Everyone laughed except the commanding officer who proceeded to chew us out on the field and ordered us to her office at ten o'clock. Since we were already in trouble and still half drunk, Libby and I decided to skip breakfast and go back to our rooms to take a nap. Besides, we had to get dressed anyway. Unfortunately, we didn't wake up until after nine o'clock. Since I overslept, I didn't report to the mess hall at seven o'clock for my scheduled training. This got added to the long list of offenses. It hadn't sunk into my head yet that I was military property and had been since I signed my enlistment contract. To me this was a vacation. I was about to find out otherwise. During my ten o'clock meeting with the commanding officer, I was given an Article 15, which is a rather severe punishment under the Uniform Code of Military Justice. For punishment, I received a suspended bust, forfeiture of half my pay for two months, extra duty in the kitchen, and was restricted to base until I transferred in a month. The commanding officer also said she was calling my future commanding officer at McGuire and apprise her of my actions. In other words, I was screwed. The extra kitchen duty consisted of reporting to the mess hall at four in the morning, five days a week, for the next three weeks to peal hundreds of potatoes. Soldiers eat a lot of potatoes. Until I had to peal hundreds of them, I didn't realize how many potatoes military personnel consumed every day. Each morning I would report to the kitchen and sit in front of three 55 gallon drums filled with potatoes. I had to peal all of them before I could leave. Needless to say, the rest of my time at Ft. Lee was uneventful. I completed my training in September and transferred to my permanent duty station, McGuire Air Force Base, N.J. This was a new duty station and a chance for a fresh start but I just wasn't quite ready to clean up my act. I don't know what happened to Libby but I heard she was subsequently discharged from the Army as "unsuitable".

Historical Marker #5: Woodstock 1969: Advertised as a Music and Arts Festival it was three days of Peace and Music held at Max Yasgur's 600 acre dairy farm in Bethel, NY, August 15-18, 1969. Over 400,000 people attended and listened to 32 performers in the rain for three days. I wish I could have attended.

I was a cook at a very large base. The chow hall served over 5000 personnel each day and never closed. I usually was assigned to the salad bar which was the largest salad bar I had ever seen. It had everything you could imagine and it took hours to prepare and prep. This salad bar covered about a third of the total food area and had over 75 items to choose from. I went to work every day on time, was in a clean uniform, looked nice and performed my duties very well. I was finally adjusting and conforming to military life but I still resented being a cook. Cooks were the bottom of the barrel. As soon as possible, I intended to retrain.

Off duty I continued to drink and stay out way too late. There weren't any bed checks anymore so we were free to come and go as we pleased. My roommates and I would go to the clubs on base two or three nights a week and pick up men. I usually drank too much and blacked out. Many nights I remember waking up by the front door of my barracks sometime in the early morning sitting on the cement and freezing cold. Apparently, the guy I had been with left me there because I was too drunk hoping the duty officer or someone else would find me and drag me into the barracks. Unfortunately, cell phones did not exist yet. At 18, I was having the time of my life. I had my own paycheck, a nice room in the barracks, plenty of good fresh food to eat, new clothes, great friends, lots of sexual attention, and freedom. One of my roommates, Kathy, had a car and we would take off to New York City once a month or so. It was only about an hour drive from the base and the USO rented us a room downtown for $15.00 a night. Remember, this was 1969, when New York City was a lot different than it is now. Times Square had all the sex shops and Greenwich Village was still in existence. If you were into drugs, Greenwich Village was the place to go. I had never seen anything like New York City at night. What a city! During the day, we went sightseeing and at night we went walking around the city. On one of our trips we took the ferry over to the Statue of Liberty. We decided to buy a soft vanilla ice cream cone and bet each other who could run up all the steps of the statue first and still have some of their ice cream left on the cone. At that time, the arm was open to the tourist and it was over a hundred steps to the top of the statue. To top it off, the stairwell was only about four feet wide. I'm glad I wasn't claustrophobic. A lot of people left the statue that day wearing some of our vanilla ice cream. Of course, none of us won the bet because all our cones were empty by the time we reached the top of the arm.

Before dark we usually took the carriage ride through Central Park and got something the eat from the street vendors while we looked in the windows of the sex shops. I had no idea what most of that stuff was but it was interesting to look at. I noticed that skuzzy older men were the primary customers of those shops. Perverts I guessed. Not far from the sex shops were the peep shows. You know the ones I'm talking about—the man pays a nominal fee to look through a small hole at a woman dancing or stripping. These skuzzy men usually left the sex shops and strolled over to the peep shows. It was fun for us to watch the action on the streets of busy New York City. Later that evening, we would wander into some of the clubs and have a drink but we always stayed together and never left with a man. We knew you could get dead in the city. And heaven help you if you actually needed a cop. There weren't many in the city and the few I saw were on foot or horseback directing traffic ignoring everything else. If you saw the original movie "The Out Of Towners" with Jack Lemmon which was filmed in New York City the same year, you get a sense of what the city was like in 1969. Today, it is cleaned up and primarily a tourist attraction. New York City used to be an adventure, now it's just a shopping spree.

During the first seven or eight months of my tour at McGuire AFB, Kathy and I took many trips other than to New York City. We also went to Atlantic City, Philadelphia, downtown Trenton, and one weekend we decided to visit George Washington Crossing National Park. Kathy, another one of my roommates, and I had dates so we packed a picnic lunch and headed out to the park. The guys decided to stop and fill a couple of coolers with beer to take with us. I didn't know at that time that it was illegal to have alcoholic beverages in a national park. I found out when the guys hung the coolers from the overhead rafters of the cooking area and said the rangers wouldn't find it up there. Since it was late October, it got dark early then it got cold, really cold. We had been wading in the river and were wet which didn't help. One of the guys tried to gather some firewood and start a fire but the wood was too wet. So the idiot started breaking up one of the park benches and lit it on fire. While we were warming up, the rangers showed and informed us that there were no visitors allowed in the park after dark, it was a federal offense to destroy park property (burning the benches), and yes they did see the cooler with beer hanging from the rafters. We all showed the rangers our military identification and begged for mercy. The two rangers showed pity on us and fined our dates (over $1000) for the offenses, told us to clean up our mess, and escorted us out of the park with a warning not to come back. That was a close call. We never went out with those three fools again or return to George Washington Crossing. What I would give to be that young, carefree and naïve one more time!

And then there was Bill . . .

I had been at McGuire less than a year when I met Bill, my first husband. We were both cooks and worked together for a short period of time. I don't know why I married him because I really never loved him. I think I loved the fact that he was in love with me and the idea of being married. Bill was in his late twenties, German decent, had been in the Air Force for about ten years, his home town was Tulsa, Oklahoma, and he came from a wealthy family. His father was a retired veterinarian. There was even a street named after him in Tulsa. Who knew his father was also a drunk? His wife would hide liquor bottles from him around the house but of course he always found them. It was just a game the two played. His father was not just a drunk, he was an abusive drunk. So was his son, Bill. Unfortunately, I didn't know this before we got married. After dating for only a couple of months, one evening Bill pulled out a fabulous diamond engagement ring and asked me to marry him. I said yes when truthfully I should have said no. I didn't know him very well. He was always on his best behavior while we were dating; the perfect gentleman. I never saw him drunk. I was usually the one that was drunk and he was taking care of me. At that time, I liked being taken care of. Bill was a senior NCO, (noncommissioned officer) an E-6 and I was a lowly E-3, so that was flattering. Usually senior NCOs don't have anything to do with junior enlisted airman. That should have been a clue that something wasn't right.

We had a very nice military wedding at the chapel on the base. Bill's parents flew up from Tulsa and helped with the wedding. This was the first time I had met them. After the reception, we drove to Reno, Nevada for our two week honeymoon. Bill had a new Cutlass Supreme with an eight track. That car was fabulous. It was a stick shift and would fly which is exactly what we did all the way from New Jersey to Nevada. The trip was fantastic. We went to the Grand Canyon, Donavan's Pass, and the Ponderosa where "Bonanza" was filmed. We even stopped in Las Vegas a couple of days and saw Elvis perform. The only thing that wasn't great was the sex. Bill was having trouble performing in bed. When he was able to perform, it lasted about five minutes and was all about him. I was young and inexperienced but I knew there had to be more than "wham, bam, thank you mam". He blamed it on the alcohol and being tired from driving but the sex never improved. Well, it was too late now.

Bill had received orders for Altus Air Force Base, OK, before we left for our honeymoon so when we returned he started processing for transfer. I received my orders about a month later and joined him in Oklahoma. During that month, Bill bought us a single wide trailer to live in and had it set up and ready to move into. The trailer furniture was alright, Spanish decor. The only thing I didn't care for were the bedrooms. All the bedroom furniture was attached to the walls so there wasn't any replacing it or rearranging it. That really bothered me. I felt like I was at camp.

Shortly after transferring to Altus, I was able to retrain as an Air Passenger/Cargo Specialist. Finally, I was away from the chow hall. I went to Wichita Falls, TX, for a short school and returned to my horrible married life at Altus. I was working nights on the flight line and Bill was working days (three on/three off) in the chow hall, hence we didn't see a lot of each other. He bought himself a Honda 750 motorcycle and drove it thereby leaving me the car. After Bill bought the motorcycle, he started spending a lot of time at bars and pool halls and didn't come home for days. When he did stumble home, he was drunk and hadn't bathed. He stunk and of course wanted sex. Having sex with a stinking drunk who couldn't perform was disgusting. Drunks reminded me of my father and I despised drunks. I finally started refusing to have sex with him. This marriage went from bad to worse. At this point, we should have agreed that this wasn't working and either sought counseling or separated. Unfortunately, that isn't what happened.

Bill and I had been married eight or nine months when I met Cris. I had gotten promoted to buck sergeant (E-4) and was in charge of the flight line night shift. Cris was an airman (E-2) who had just completed his "A" school and had recently arrived at his permanent duty station, Altus. He was the cutest, sexiest guy I had ever met. It was instant lust for me. Cris was from Ponca City, Oklahoma, six foot tall, muscular, light brown hair, green eyes, and 19 years old, a couple of years younger than me. I later found out his parents worked for Conoco in Ponca City, and were looking to retire in about ten years. Cris said he had been attending a junior college when he got his draft notice, so he joined the Air Force to avoid the draft. Since I was his supervisor, it was also my job to train him so we were together all night five nights a week. Needless to say, after a couple of months we got real close. I wanted to jump in bed with Cris from the moment I first saw him but I kept it professional for several months. It was hard being unhappily married and not cheating. Eventually I asked Cris over to the trailer for a drink and to watch a football game. Bill was on his three days off and I hadn't seen or heard from him in two days. After having a couple of drinks, Cris and I starting making out on the sofa in the living room. I knew what I was doing was wrong but I couldn't help myself. Both of us were afraid Bill would come home so it only went as far as kissing and touching. Sure enough we heard the sound of Bill's motorcycle pull in next to the trailer. Bill recognized Cris' car and charged into the trailer demanding what the hell was going on. He then came at Cris who was quickly making his way to the front door a few feet away. Cris ran out the door, jumped into his Chevy SS and took off before a confrontation could erupt. Unfortunately, that left Bill and I standing there staring at each other. Bill as usual had been drinking and smelled and looked like he had been up all night. He turned and went into the bedroom looking for the .22 caliber handgun he kept in the nightstand. I had hidden the gun earlier that week because of the tension between us. Maybe I predicted and wanted a confrontation. After he couldn't find the gun in the bedroom, Bill came back into the living room and the beating began. He asked where the gun was and grabbed me by my long blond hair then began dragging me down the hallway to the bedroom. Along the way he was slapping me in the face and asking if I thought he was an idiot and calling me a whore. He also reminded me he was a former member of Hells Angels and could have me killed with one phone call. Bill then ordered me to get undressed and forced me to have sex with him. Having sex with a drunk is disgusting. They stink, they sweat like a pig, and they can't perform but keep trying. Eventually, Bill fell asleep or passed out and I got partially dressed, grabbed my purse and keys and took off like a bat out of hell. I actually left the trailer without shoes or a coat and it was late fall. I went to the transient barracks on base where I stayed for several weeks. The next day I filed a domestic abuse complaint against Bill with the on base police. They took photos of my black eye and bruised face and told me not to go back to the trailer without a police escort. The complaint I filed against Bill was presented to his commanding officer that afternoon and he was escorted to the trailer for some of his belongings then ordered confined to a barracks room on base. He was busted one rank and ordered to attend alcohol and psychological counseling. The next week I was told he slashed his wrists in an attempt to commit suicide. A few days later, Bill's mother contacted me requesting permission to enter the trailer in order to retrieve the rest of Bill's personal belongings. Since Bill was still confined and I did not think his mother was a threat to me, I agreed to meet her at the trailer. We didn't talk much. She told me Bill was in counseling and would be transferred to a different duty station in the near future. When we were in the kitchen packing a few things, she slapped me in the face and asked me how I could do this to her son. I never expected this and never saw it coming. While I was recovering, she grabbed the rest of her packed items and left. And that was the end of Bill and my one year marriage. I sent him the divorce papers to sign a couple of weeks later and he did so without incident. I got the trailer, all the belongings inside it, and the car. I never saw or heard from Bill again. I do hope he managed to salvage his military career and retire. I always felt badly about my actions that provoked our confrontation. I kept three things as mementos, an 8"x10" black and white wedding photo, my diamond from my engagement ring which I had remounted, and a Sunbeam electric mixer that his mother was holding in one hand as she slapped me with the other.

All about Cris . . .

During my divorce, Cris and I didn't see each other. We both thought we should let things cool off for awhile. Our commanding officer transferred Cris to the day shift after he found out about the incident at the trailer with Bill. After a couple of months, we picked up where we left off. I started seeing Cris almost every day. I had my freedom back and was enjoying every minute of it. As I said earlier, I had long blonde hair at the time and was quite a sex pot at 5'4", 120 lbs, and very fit. I started dressing provocatively again—short leather skirts, tight sweaters, boots, lots of make up, fish net nylons, and plenty of jewelry. I don't know why other than it felt good. I was hot and enjoyed flaunting it for a change. Cris couldn't keep his hands off of me. The sex between us was explosive. I had my first orgasm with Cris and I absolutely adored him. I remember him saying after I climaxed "see, you can have your cake and eat it too". After a few months, we decided it was time to meet each others parents starting with his so we took a few days leave and drove up to Ponca City. During this first visit Cris' parents, Sam and Jean were cordial but not very warm and they asked a lot of questions. I got the feeling right away that they did not particularly care for me. Now I understand that they were only trying to protect their only son from what they perceived a big mistake. In other words, I wasn't exactly who they had in mind as a mate for their son. My recent divorce stuck in their craw along with the fact that I was about two years older and in the military. Cris said they would eventually come around but they never did. Since he was close to his parents, particularly his mother, they became a wedge in our relationship. Cris later told me that they had ordered him to stop seeing me but of course he didn't. Instead we started spending more and more time together. It was like two moths being drawn toward the same light bulb.

The following month, we drove to Texas to see my mom and her new husband, Ray. We had a great time and enjoyed the short trip. One embarrassing incident happened that I just have to tell on myself. Cris and I went out drinking one night and I got totally wasted on Singapore Slings. I started ripping off my clothes in the car and tried to get Cris to pull over and have sex. Of course he didn't but might have if I hadn't started throwing up. When we got back to mom's house, I had to really use the bathroom. I was so drunk I didn't raise the toilet lid and took a crap on top of it. Then apparently I raised the lid when I finished thereby sticking the lid (with all the crap on it) to the toilet tank. That is exactly how mom found it the next morning when she got up to take her morning pee. I have never drunk Singapore Slings again. While we were there, Cris and I slept together in the same bed which is something we didn't do at his parents' house. Jean assigned me the extra bedroom at the far end of the house and put Cris on the living room sofa. When I got up in the middle of the night, Cris was never on the sofa. He was usually in his parents' bedroom talking to them with the door shut. This should have been a big red flag for things to come.

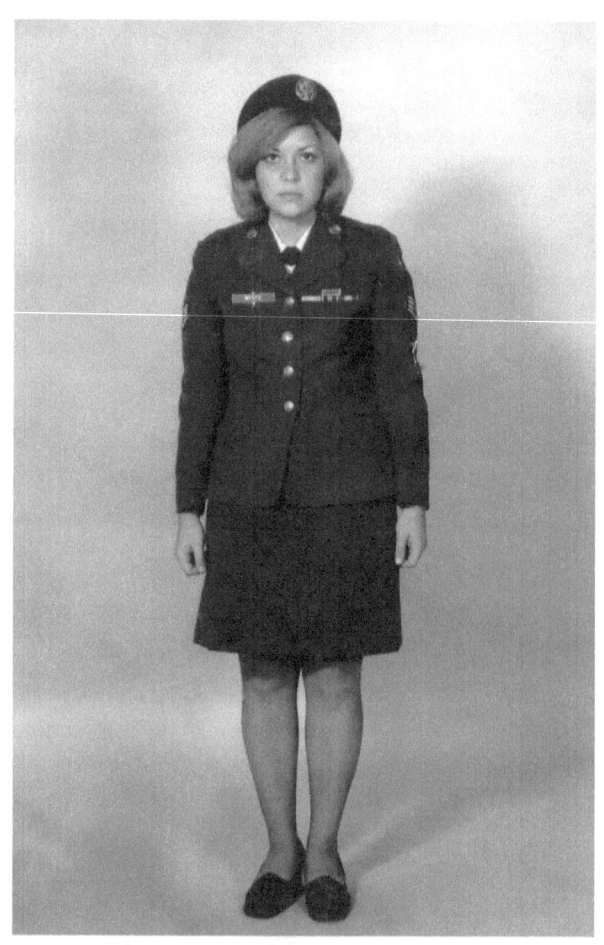

Me, in my Air Force uniform as a SSgt, 1973

CHAPTER 6

True Love—Not So Much (Age 23-27)

In the spring of 1972, I was promoted to E-5 (SSgt). I had only been in the Air Force two years and eleven months. This was record time because I had fantastic evaluations and aced the written tests for promotion. I guess I had finally cleaned up my act. With this rapid promotion came an unexpected opportunity, being nominated for drill instructor. I submitted my paperwork and photo and waited for a response. I was so physically fit it was ridiculous. I could do 50-60 pushups, 150 plus sit-ups, run the mile and a half in about ten minutes and looked like a model from a fitness magazine. While I was waiting for a response to my drill instructor request, a treaty was signed with North Viet Nam ending the war at the end of the year. Many active duty personnel were offered a three month early out in order to reduce the number of troops on active duty who were no longer needed since the war was over. The draft ended a few months later. My four year enlistment was up in May 1973, however in January of that year I was offered the early out and agreed to take it. I was discharged from active duty on February 13, 1973. The primary reason I agreed to accept the early discharge was because I was pregnant with Cris' child. I withdrew my request to become a drill instructor. At that time, pregnant female members were not allowed to remain on active duty. A lot has changed in that respect since 1973.

Over the past year, Cris and I had made many trips to his parents' house in Ponca City in hopes of gaining their approval because we wanted to get married. That approval never came so in December of 1972, I decided to stop taking my birth control pills and was pregnant in less than two months. I really thought it would take longer since I had been on the pill for over four years. When I told Cris I was pregnant, I could tell he was both happy and scared. He was only 20 years old and this was a huge responsibility. This was a selfish and unwise decision on my part. Trapping a man into marriage almost always dooms the marriage to failure. At that time, Oklahoma's law required the male be 21 years old to marry without parental consent. Therefore, Cris took leave and we eloped to Livingston, Alabama where we were married. I was now Cris' military dependent. Upon discharge from the military, the member gets one paid relocation move. Since Cris was due for transfer soon, we decided to have the military move my trailer to Texas for my mother to use while we were gone. That summer Cris received his transfer orders to Anderson Air Force Base, Guam. It was a three year tour since he was taking his family with him. Cris and I lived in a small apartment off base in Altus until our beautiful daughter, Dannielle, was born in late September. I spent the summer pregnant in very hot southern Oklahoma with no air conditioning. It was a miserable summer. I gained over 25 lbs. and my ankles swelled up the size of grapefruits making it difficult to walk. My favorite meal was slightly browned hamburger patties (virtually raw) with over easy eggs cooked in the same skillet with a piece of toast. Cris was working as a loadmaster and was away from home about 75% of the time. I remember sitting on the front porch most of the day with my feet in an ice bucket and wet rags around my neck trying to stay cool. Inside that tiny apartment was like an oven even with the windows open. Dannielle was born the last week of September 1973 at the base hospital. I remember when my water broke and I woke Cris up to take me to the hospital. I was so relieved to finally be in labor and end the torture of being very pregnant. I was in labor over 14 hours, had 21 stitches and a hemorrhoid since the doctors insisted on a natural birth. Cris was in the delivery room and watched the birth of our daughter. I cussed him and bit his arm during contractions. My body was not built to have children. After this delivery from hell, I decided one child was enough for me. Dannielle would be an only child. Cris' mother, Jean drove down and stayed with us a few days after Dannielle and I were discharged from the hospital. I guess she meant well but honestly she wasn't much help particularly since we didn't get along very well.

Now that the baby was here, it was all about the three of us making the transfer to Guam. We agreed Dannielle and I would stay with my mother for about a month while Cris found us a place to live on Guam. Dannielle and I boarded the plane in Dallas and took off for Guam after Thanksgiving; she was just two months old. That was the longest flight I had endured in my life. Traveling half way around the world with a small baby was horrific to say the least. The flight attendants would not heat her bottles for me so she was forced to drink cold formula the entire 20 hour flight. Anyone who has had a baby knows that cold milk gives a baby gas and they cry which is exactly what happened. Dannielle didn't sleep more than a couple of hours the entire flight which means neither did I. Both of us were exhausted by the time we finally landed on Guam.

Guam is an island 35 miles long and 7 miles wide out in the middle of the Atlantic roughly seven hours flying time from Hawaii, across the International Date Line, not far from the Philippines. In other words, it's a rock out in the middle of nowhere. It is the arm pit of the Universe. In 1973, Guam had no real telephone service, no air conditioning, only one main paved road, no movie theatres, no restaurants, only one local television station, and lots of old World War II Quonset huts. Basically, there was nothing appealing about Guam. The apartment Cris had rented for us was a small duplex located about five or six miles from the base. We lived among the locals who spoke only broken English. Anything we needed had to be obtained from the base. Our apartment consisted of three rooms and a small bath which only had a shower—no bathtub to bathe Dannielle. It was always hot and humid in Guam. It rained every day at 3 p.m., and there was no air conditioning, only a water cooler window fan which caused everything in the apartment to mold. I developed serious sinus problems because of the mold in our apartment. You had two choices: mold or suffocate from the heat and humidity. One thing that apartment had plenty of was large flying roaches. Those things were three inches long and they lived off of roach spray. They would attack me at night when I got up to go to the bathroom. One night one of those monsters attacked me and I jumped on the bathroom sink to get away from it and wound up ripping the sink off the wall. Cris was ticked because he had to fix it. You couldn't kill those suckers even by stepping on them. I had never seen a cockroach as hearty as these in my entire life and still haven't. Since we didn't ship a car to Guam, Cris bought a used orange Toyota for us to drive while on the "rock". It was pretty pathetic but at least it ran.

The years on Guam were pretty horrible. I detested Guam. Cris was only an E-3 at the time and his military pay ($650 a month) was barely enough to live on. I wasn't working now so we were poor and living pay check to pay check. After about a year, Cris got promoted to E-4 and we moved to a larger apartment which was a little nicer but it still didn't have a telephone, air conditioning, or washer/dryer. At least it didn't have the monster roaches. Cris of course was away from home most of the time so Dannielle and I spent a lot of time at the beach. I liked sitting on the beach early in the morning and late in the evening because the sound of the waves were soothing and the air off the ocean was cool and refreshing. I would put Dannielle in diapers with a plastic cover on the outside and let her play in the water and mud on the beach. She started walking when she was nine months old and was potty trained when she was seven months old. I had to potty train her at that young age because she kept pulling her Pampers off and tearing the stuffing out. Dannielle did not like wearing diapers. She was a beautiful, remarkable baby and a constant companion. When I got out of the Air Force and became a dependent I had no idea what that really meant. It meant that I gave up my identity and depended on someone else (Cris) to support me. I was simply Mrs. Cris King. I had no identity, no source of income, was completely isolated, had no friends, and was fat and ugly. In other words, I had "no pot, no window". I hadn't lost the weight I had gained during pregnancy, so once again in my life I was fat and ugly. Cris would give me an allowance each week, $20, like I was a child. It wasn't long before we were arguing over the lack of money and our marriage started to crumble. The more we argued, the less Cris was home. We eventually stopped talking to each other then we stopped having sex. I went to see a Guamanian attorney seeking a separation from Cris. He told me I was damaged goods since I had a child that no other man would want to raise and advised me to patch things up with Cris. I more or less accepted my fate and starting making an effort to save the marriage until I accidently found two letters from other women not on Guam that he was seeing. We had been on the rock about two years and I was on base and decided to check our post office box. Cris usually checked the box so I guess he felt comfortable giving that address to other women. Cris was having multiple affairs! I'm sure there were more than the two I stumbled upon. No wonder he wasn't interested in me sexually. When I confronted him with the letters, he snatched them out of my hand and told me to mind my own business. It was too late—I had read them. After yet another argument, Cris packed a couple of bags and moved to the barracks. This was the beginning of the end. Even though he eventually moved back home, we both felt the strain of this failing marriage. Unknown to me at the time, Cris was calling his parents on a regular basis from the base. This becomes an important issue a few months later.

Around six months or so before the end of our tour on Guam, the island was hit with a monsoon, a 7.6 earthquake, and several tornadoes all in a twenty four hour period. Cris of course wasn't home. Dannielle was asleep on the living room floor and I was trying to seal the windows to keep the driving rain out. It was a loosing battle because the wind was blowing over 75 miles per hour and it was pouring buckets. In the mist of all of this chaos, the floor started moving, the dishes began rattling and the pictures started falling off the walls. I hadn't heard any warnings or reports of violent weather so I was completely ignorant regarding the true danger Dannielle and I were in. We lived on the second floor so I knew I needed to get Dannielle and myself out of there as soon as possible because the building had started swaying. I had never experienced a monsoon, earthquake or tornado so I was pretty dumbfounded as to what to do next. I had wrapped Dannielle in a blanket and grabbed her diaper bag on the way out of the apartment and was just standing in the middle of the parking lot when a neighbor pulled me into her one story apartment. Cris showed up in the orange Toyota a few minutes later and we went to one of the new high rise hotels downtown to wait out the storm and after shocks. We were there three days. The monsoon had done tremendous damage and the earthquake had torn up roads, runways, and buildings. I don't know the total causality count, but several people died on base from heart attacks or from falling into the craters left by the earthquake. I guess we were lucky we weren't injured and made it off that rock alive. It took months to clean up the damage to the island and I later learned that one of the small islands surrounding Guam disappeared off the map.

A few months later, Cris received his transfer orders to Valdosta Air Force Base, Georgia. We had been trying to reconcile and I thought it was going fairly well. Apparently that was just all smoke and mirrors. Shortly after we arrived at Valdosta and had settled in, Cris' new car arrived. I didn't even know he had ordered a car from the military exchange before leaving Guam. His parents, whom he had been calling from the base, had helped him purchase a new Chevy SS. One afternoon while Dannielle and I had been out grocery shopping (in the orange Toyota), Cris had left to pick up his new car. When I returned home and asked him where the new car came from he informed me his parents had helped him buy it in exchange for getting rid of me. My mouth hit the floor and we starting arguing about his deception. The entire time I was talking he was gathering up Dannielle and my belongings and throwing them outside. He then suggested that I get anything else I wanted and load it in the car because our marriage was over. We had just gotten back our income tax refund, a little over $400. Cris handed me half of it and said "go take a fucking permanent vacation to your mothers". After a few minutes, he said I was moving too slow so he opened the front door and started pitching clothes, pots and pans, Dannielle's baby things, and even an ironing board out on the front lawn. Then he threw me the keys to the orange Toyota which had no heat or air conditioning, said good bye and slammed the door. As tragic as this seems, he actually did me a huge favor. I would not be the person I am today if he had not thrown me out and forced me to take care of myself as well as Dannielle, who was only two years old. Thank you Cris! I haven't talked to him for over twenty six years but I bet he's still a momma's boy. She wore the pants in that family.

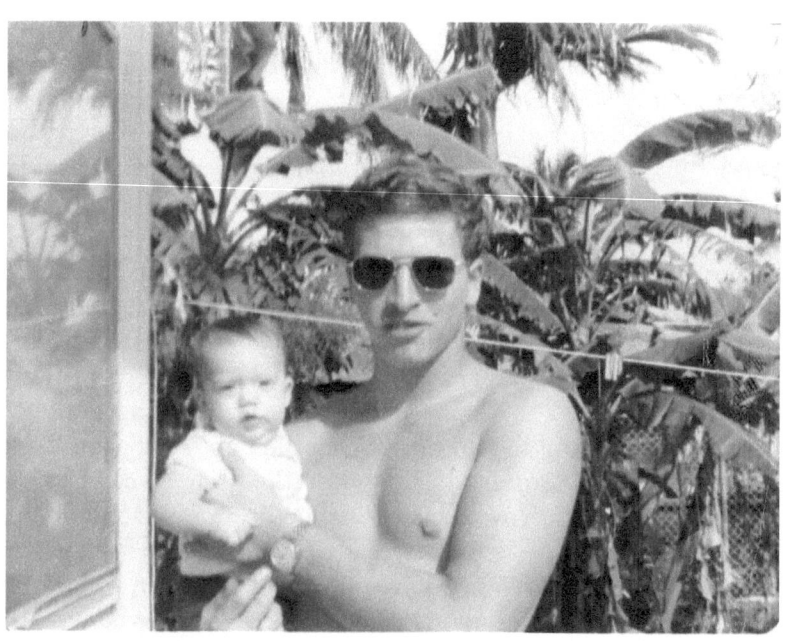

Cris and Dannielle in Guam, 1974

CHAPTER 7

Starting Over Plus One (Age 28-31)

Here I was once again, "no pot, no window"! It was the spring of 1976, and I was homeless with all my possessions crammed in a ratty old orange Toyota that had no heat or air conditioning. Additionally, it wasn't just me I had to take care of now, I had a two year old daughter that depended on me completely for her well being. The only money I had was the two hundred dollar income tax refund so stopping at a hotel for the night during the drive from Georgia to Texas wasn't an option. I had called mom before I left Georgia and told her I was on my way. She was less than enthusiastic about me returning home under these circumstances. Mom made it clear that I needed to find a job and move out as soon as possible and she wasn't babysitting. I was devastated and felt abandoned and betrayed by Cris. I had no idea how I was going to survive and be able to support Dannielle since I had no viable skills or college in 1976. I drove straight through from Valdosta to Tyler only stopping for gas, short rest breaks, and to take care of Dannielle.

Dannielle and I stayed with mom for a couple of months until I finally found a job at Regan's Department Store in Tyler as a credit clerk. Shortly thereafter, I was able to find a cheap one bedroom, partially furnished apartment not far from work. Mom and Ray (who had recently married) were also living in an apartment in Tyler and renting out the trailer I had given them. The trailer was parked in a low rent trailer park in a suburb outside Tyler. I told mom I needed the trailer and to let me know when the current tenants lease expired. The trailer was furnished and almost paid for. As much as I hated the thought of moving back into that trailer, it was a lot better than what I had now—pretty much nothing.

The cheap apartment we moved into had a bed, a torn up sofa, and a card table which served as a dining table. I couldn't afford to buy any furniture so

Dannielle and I slept together on the full bed and scrounged milk crates to use as tables. Mom had an old television she gave us along with a fan since as usual there was no air conditioning. The place was pretty much a dump but it was a roof over our heads. I hadn't heard from Cris since I left Georgia almost three months earlier, so I called him at his work on base, gave him my address, and asked him to send some money for Dannielle. He agreed to send money but of course he didn't. I didn't get a dime out of him until I filed for a divorce and called his commanding officer eight months later. His commanding officer ordered him to send money or face disciplinary action. If Cris hadn't been in the military, I probably wouldn't have gotten any support from him. I don't understand why men think they don't have a responsibility to support their children after the marriage is over. Raising a child as a single parent is difficult enough without fighting to get a few dollars child support every month.

Trying to cope with life everyday was very difficult. I was still fat, had coke bottle lens glasses, ragged clothes from Goodwill, and virtually no self esteem. I felt like a bag of garbage that had gotten thrown out for the trash man to pick up. I had gone from a fairly attractive young woman with a promising career in the Air Force to this in less than four years. I contemplated suicide many times that first year Cris and I were separated. The only thing that stopped me was the thought of who would raise Dannielle. My guess was Cris' parents since they had wanted to adopt her when we separated. I despised Cris' parents and there was no way the two of them were going to have custody of Dannielle. As a coping mechanism I started drinking quite a bit usually after work. In other words, I never called off work because I was too drunk or hung over to get up on Monday morning. Anything to get rid of the loneliness and pain I felt. Maybe secretly I was hoping I would overdose on alcohol—just pass out and never wake up. I remember I bought a FM radio to listen to and kept a bottle of Jim Beam in the house for after work. I would come home from work, feed Dannielle and give her a bath, watch a little television with her, and then after I put her to bed I would drag out the Jim Beam and turn on the radio. Those were very lonely days. It wasn't long before I realized that Cris had moved on with his life and didn't care about me or his daughter. I really began to hate him.

After Cris signed the divorce papers, I received $75 dollars a month child support like clockwork every month on the 15th. For awhile he sent Dannielle birthday and Christmas presents but that dwindled the older she got. I took Dannielle to Oklahoma a few times to visit Cris' parents but they offered no financial help either. The child support from Cris paid for the babysitter while I was at work and little of anything else. Financially I was at my wits end. I started drawing WIC and food stamps to help make ends meet. There were a lot of nights that we ate macaroni and cheese or peanut butter sandwiches and called it dinner.

Over the next year I slowly pulled myself out of poverty. I slowed down on the drinking, managed to lose a few pounds and bought us some new clothes. I also went to the optometrist and got a pair of hard contact lenses. Contact lenses had just come on the market in the form of hard lenses only. At first, I could only wear them two hours a day and had to work up to ten hours over a period of time. I couldn't believe how much better I looked without those coke bottle glasses. I was slowly regaining my self esteem but I was still poor. I had accepted the fact that Cris was never coming back and unless I wanted to continue living my life with "no pot and no window" I needed to make some changes. I had a daughter to support and I wanted so much more for her. No one in my family had ever obtained a college degree but with any luck, I might be the first. I had the Viet Nam Veterans G.I. Bill and decided to use it. I applied to Tyler Junior College in the fall, passed the SAT, and started with two basic core classes two nights a week. Since I couldn't afford a babysitter while I went to school, I usually took Dannielle with me. The instructors said they didn't mind as long as she was quite. I never quit taking classes. I realized the only way out of poverty was education. Additionally, I vowed I would never again depend on anyone financially except myself to take care of Dannielle and me. I wasn't going to look for the perfect frog all my life like my mother had.

In the spring of 1977, my old trailer became available so I cleaned it up and Dannielle and I moved in. It needed some new mattresses, a dining table and chairs, and a very through cleaning. I went to Sears and bought a stereo, some new linens and a few decorator items trying to make the old trailer feel homey. Mom was working nights at a Certified gas station at the time so I asked if I could work with her one or two nights a week for a little extra cash. Now I had a toddler, a full time job, a part time job, and was attending college two nights a week. Dannielle tagged along with me to my part time job at the gas station. In 1977, nights at gas stations were relatively safe and she played in the store while mom and I worked. That August, Elvis Presley died of a drug over dose while sitting on his toilet at Graceland. I was crushed when I heard the news.

Historical Marker #6: The King of Rock and Roll was dead. Elvis Presley was dead! Why? For drugs? This was absurd. I'll never forget the date, August 13, 1977. The first movie I remember seeing was "Jail House Rock" (1957) at a drive-in theatre in Marshall. My father took all of the family to see Elvis' new movie. Elvis once said "ambition is a dream with a V8 engine". How True! In 1980, I visited Graceland in Memphis and saw Elvis' and his twin brother Aaron's grave. I guess in some ways Elvis will never die.

In 1978, the disco era arrived. "Saturday Night Fever" with John Travolta and the music of the Bee Gees went down in history. I still have the albums I bought in 1978 of "Saturday Night Fever" and "Staying Alive" by the Bee Gees. "Dirty Dancing" with Patrick Swayze had just come on the scene as well.

I started saving enough money out of my pay to allow myself to go to a disco a couple of times a month. Discos reenergized you. They made you feel good again. All the lights and the people dancing were magnificent. What a great time that was!

Even though I was working full time and part time, I never seemed to have enough money. One winter Anne had to buy groceries for Dannielle and me on her credit card in order for us to have food on the table until payday rolled around again. I really appreciated that hundred dollars worth of food. The struggle for survival was getting to be too much. There had to be something better. After some deliberation, I decided to join the military again. The Air Force only offered me pay grade of E-2 as a hospital corpsman, so I declined their offer since I had gotten out as an E-5. I contacted the Navy and they offered me (as a reservist) E-4, Yeoman. A Yeoman is equivalent to an administrative assistant. I gladly accepted their offer and started drilling as a Navy Reservist in Tyler in the winter of 1977. My pay for one drill weekend a month was slightly over a hundred dollars. That check every month meant so much—food on the table. Anne usually kept Dannielle while I drilled and she had a great time playing with Anne's two kids, Paul and Mikelle. Paul was about three years older and Mikelle was a year younger. What a trio they made.

I guess I need to regress and tell you that Anne had divorced her first husband Victor not long after his discharge from the Air Force. Not long after her divorce, while I was in Guam, she met and married Mikel. Mikelle is Mikel's daughter. Paul and Mikelle never really got along. They fought like cats and dogs and still do. Anne met Mikel while she was working at one of the local hospitals in Tyler as a lab technician. Mikel was driving an ambulance at the time. They bought a double wide mobile home and parked it on Mikel's parents' property a few miles outside the city limits of Tyler. Mikel was a very disturbed individual. He drank and used drugs on a regular basis. When he was messed up, he became abusive usually toward Paul or Anne. I never knew what she saw in him because they were like oil and water since Anne had always been religious. Mikel lost his ambulance driving job when he was transporting a seven year old girl to the hospital higher than a kite and ran a red light without sounding his horn on the ambulance. Consequently, he hit a vehicle in the intersection and as a result of that accident the little girl died before reaching the hospital. Mikel was charged criminally and sued by the little girl's parents. Things at Anne's home got pretty bad. On more than one occasion the police were called to their mobile home for a domestic disturbance. Anne eventually decided she had had enough and filed for divorce and Mikel moved into his parents' home during the separation. Mikel was eventually committed to Rusk Mental Hospital for about a year and Anne hoped he would clean up his act and get off the drugs. Upon release, Mikel returned home and found part time employment. Unfortunately he was never able to get off the alcohol and drugs. The last year of his poor miserable life he sat out in his shack he had built out back and drank his booze, smoked his weed, and snorted his coke with his ZZ Top music blaring. In my opinion, Mikel has a horrible husband and not much of a father. One summer afternoon in 1979, Mikel took a pistol out of the glove box of his pickup truck and blew his brains out. He was sitting in his truck in front of their trailer at the mailbox when he killed himself. Mikel was a very troubled man. After he shot himself, his body fell over the steering wheel causing the horn to blow. Anne came out to see what was wrong and found him dead with his brains splattered all over the windshield. Not long after Mikel's death, his mother sold their trailer and all its contents while Anne was away from home for a few days. Unfortunately, since this left Anne with nothing, she was forced into the "no pot, no window" plight for over three years. Today Mikel is six feet under and Anne is retired drawing his social security survivor benefits. Mikel killed himself before their divorce was final. Karma caught up with Mikel and you simply can't out run Karma!

I might as well bring you up to date with Betty too. While I was at boot camp, she got drunk and wrecked my precious Mustang. Mom told me she was drunk and ran into a tree totaling the car. I was really ticked off and didn't talk to her for a long time. I had planned on taking leave before reporting to McGuire and driving the Mustang up to New Jersey. Well, forget that. I didn't have another car for over two years. In 1971, Betty met and married her first husband Pete. They bought a house in Athens about 35 miles from Tyler heading toward Waco. Pete worked for Magnavox and Betty was a bookkeeper and seasonal tax preparer. Over the next three years they had two children, Chris and Tonya. Two perfectly beautiful kids—blonde hair and green eyes. Chris is about a year older than Dannielle and Tonya is a year or so younger. Their marriage was good for roughly ten years then it completely disintegrated. But this is 1978, and all is well. I didn't know it at the time but a storm was brewing on the horizon. Mom and Ray bought a home in the same subdivision in 1977. I can only imagine how thrilled Pete and Betty were to have mom living a few doors down.

My first summer drill in the Navy Reserves was two weeks at NAS Dallas in Grand Prairie, a suburb of Dallas. The two weeks were fun and provided a short break from everything else—my other jobs and school. I stayed in the barracks on base and drove back to Tyler on the weekends. Dannielle stayed with Anne and seemed to enjoy her time with Paul and Mikelle. After this first summer drill I knew I wanted to go back on active duty and started inquiring how this might become a reality. The administrative personnel I worked with while at NAS Dallas told me about an active duty program for reservist called TAR (temporary active duty reservist). It would require me to sign a one year active duty contract which could be renewed if the billet was still available.

This sounded perfect. I could go on active duty, one year at a time and not have to move. Once I returned to my normal drill weekends in Tyler, I asked my supervisor to check into a billet for me, either in Tyler or Dallas. A couple of months later he told me a billet at the Navy Recruiting Office in Dallas was going to be available in about six months if I wanted to apply for it. Of course I did. I was truly sick and tired of working my butt off and not seeming to be getting anywhere. The only thing I was really interested in right then was college and the Navy. I decided to submit my request for the TAR position and hope I was selected. At this time, I had completed roughly a year and a half of college and was still enrolled. As it turned out, this was one of the reasons I was selected for the billet. There were 15 or more reservists who also applied for the position but I was the lucky one who was selected. Finally, I was digging myself out of poverty.

Since I anticipated working in Dallas in the near future, I decided to move the ratty old trailer one more time. I selected a nice trailer park in Seagoville. Seagoville is about a 45 minute drive from Tyler and about 25 minutes from downtown Dallas. Perfect! It took one day to prep the trailer for the move, one day to actually move it and another two days to put in on blocks, wrap the water pipes with heat insulation, and put up the underpinning. After all of that was done, I still had to unpack everything and clean. Basically, it was a week of moving. Dannielle and I stayed with Anne for a few days during the move. This was shortly before Mikel's suicide and I really got to see what an ass Mikel was while I was there. Anne was still drinking and smoking (she later quit both) so we sat up, had a few drinks and talked. This is when I realized how miserable she was and that this marriage was also ending badly in the near future. I felt sorry for Anne. She never could find the right man either. They all seemed to be assholes and idiots these days.

Speaking of assholes and idiots, shortly before I went back on active duty and started working in Dallas, Anne convinced me to go with her to visit our father. I had not seen him or heard from him in 20 years and did not want to make the trip but I decided to appease Anne and go. So, we loaded the three kids, Paul, Mikelle, and Dannielle in the car and took off. My father, James, was living in Jefferson, a small city not far from Marshall, with his wife of several decades, Lucille. They were living in a ratty rented house out in the middle of nowhere. Their primary source of income was Lucille's social security check. My father had been using aliases since the late '50's when he ran over a man with his car (killing him) in Houston while he was driving drunk. There was a warrant out for his arrest for vehicular homicide stemming from this incident so he changed his name to Stetson, like the hat, and started working for cash only. He never used his social security number since law enforcement would have been able to find him by tracing any activity on it. I'm sure 20 years later there were several warrants out on him for various assaults as well since he frequented bars and bragged about instigating fights at the bars. My father was a real piece of work. The first thing he did when we got to his house was offer us a glass of his home brewed wine. As it turned out, he was fermenting a batch in the bath tub and took us in the bathroom to show us his brew. Anne and I of course declined his offer for a drink but he was steadily sucking the mess down. Paul, Mikelle, and Dannielle were outside playing on a swing set thank goodness because he was getting drunker by the minute. It wasn't long before he was calling me Martha Faye, my mother's name, and telling me he should have cut my throat or blew my brains out when he had the chance. Well, that was our clue to leave. Anne and I stood up to say good bye and he grabbed me by the arm and pushed me down a small flight of stairs. It scared my to death but I wasn't seriously hurt. Lucille pulled him off of me and Anne and I ran for the door. We grabbed the kids and sped off. That was the last time I saw my father. He died in 2000 of lung cancer and you got it, I did not go to the funeral. I know there was a special place in Hell waiting for him! My father abandoned us in 1958, and never showed any remorse. How did he think mom, who only had an eighth grade education and no viable job skills, was going to support three young children? Apparently he just didn't care. His actions instigated the "no pot, no window" cycle that I have fought all my life.

The winter of 1978-79 was brutal. I was still driving that old orange Toyota with no heat. It was minus five with snow, ice, and sleet that winter in Seagoville. Without a heater, you can't defrost the windows—hello. I resorted to pouring lukewarm water on the windshield and chipping and beating the ice off with an old pot and a huge butcher knife. I would wrap Dannielle up in three or four layers of clothes and drive to the babysitters' house and then to work. By the time I got to work an hour later if I made it, I was frozen. Consequently, I had bronchitis twice that winter and I was constantly taking Dannielle to the doctor with ear infections. Thank goodness she was still a military dependent since Cris was still on active duty and her medical expenses were paid for by the government. I didn't have any medical insurance at the time and couldn't afford to keep going to the doctor, so I stayed sick that winter. It was horrible not having medical or dental insurance and trying to stay well enough to continue working. I couldn't wait for the position at Dallas to become available where I could return to active duty. Being on active duty meant I had medical insurance again and could see a military doctor at NAS Dallas if I needed to. It also meant I could get my teeth cleaned and checked. None of that had been done since I left active duty in 1973. Also, by going back on active duty I would only have that one job and my pay would almost triple. Finally, this was a way to break out of the poverty cycle. If by chance I did manage to complete college and receive my degree I wouldn't have to scratch and claw every day just to survive. I could say good bye to the "no pot, no window" spiral.

Before I started my active duty tour in Dallas, I had one more two week summer drill. This time the Navy sent me to San Diego to load ships with their necessary rations before deploying. I'm sorry but I really did not like California. There were too many weird people who didn't really seem to care about anyone but themselves. New York City was weird but in a fun way. San Diego was just plain weird. In the lawns around the ship yard there were signs that said "Sailors and Dogs Stay off the Grass". How insulting! I even ventured to Los Angeles and San Francisco and didn't care for those cities either. The only thing I liked was riding the cable cars in San Francisco. Of course Anne kept Dannielle while I was gone. If it hadn't been for Anne's help by keeping Dannielle during these years I would not have been able to go back into the Navy—reserve or active duty. Shortly after returning from San Diego, I decided it was time to start looking for a new car. The old orange Toyota had to go. As it turned out I bought another Toyota. I decided to buy a brand new blue Toyota Corolla. I had been on active duty less than one month when I made the first real major purchase in my 27 years on this planet—a new car. The smell of a new car is fabulous.

Working at the Navy Recruiting Office in Dallas was fun. I enjoyed being back on active duty and around other military people. We all dressed alike, talked the same military language, had similar experiences, and most of all you always knew who was in charge. Being in the military is like having your family around you. Also, everybody is upfront and direct with you. In other words, no cut throat games like in the private sector. I was assigned to the commanding officer as his personal secretary. I could type over 80 words a minute on the IBM Selectric typewriter which pleased him very much. My days consisted of getting him coffee and sometimes lunch, typing his correspondence, filing, answering the telephone, and whatever else he needed done that day. I made a few friends at the office, Tom and Lydia, and went out with them occasionally after work. One of my neighbors at the trailer park, Ruth, was watching Dannielle while I worked and didn't mind her staying a little longer if I decided to go out. Life was good and returning to a somewhat routine and normal rhythm. I didn't miss Cris anymore. I had finally moved on emotionally. I was still lonely, but I kept busy and learned to enjoy quite time by myself. It was 1979, and I had been on my own three years.

Things were rolling along nicely until one spring Saturday morning I woke up with a headache and when I tried to stand up to go get some coffee and Tylenol, I couldn't. My knees gave out and I fell on the floor hitting my head on the side of the dresser. I was so dizzy I felt drunk but I hadn't been drinking the night before. I had no idea what was wrong with me but I knew I needed help so I crawled from the back bedroom to the front door, opened it and started yelling for Ruth. As soon as that fresh air hit me and I took a couple of deep breaths I begin to feel better. Ruth heard my yelling after a few minutes and came to her door to see what was wrong. I yelled "help" and she ran over and helped me get up and walking and got Dannielle out of the trailer. It was cold outside so we all went to her trailer, had some coffee, warmed up and tried to decide what was wrong. Ruth suggested we might need to go to the doctor and get checked out. As soon as I was able to function, I drove Dannielle and me to the clinic in town. The doctor on duty said it was carbon monoxide poisoning and gave us a little fresh oxygen. He said we were lucky to be alive and explained how faulty furnaces emit carbon monoxide into the air without it being detected since it is odorless. The doctor told me to turn off the furnace until I got it repaired and air out the trailer before I went back inside. Well this was special. Not only did Dannielle and I almost die, I didn't have the money to repair the furnace. Now I guess we would freeze to death. That ratty trailer was ten years old and as far as I knew the furnace had never been serviced and the homeowners' insurance had expired years ago. Ruth and Anne came to our rescue and bought or loaned me a couple of electric heaters until I could afford to get the furnace repaired or replaced. The following month I had a repairman come out and thank goodness he was able to repair the furnace instead of replacing it but the bill was still close to $500 dollars. That was one paycheck. Active duty military get paid twice a month—on the 1st and the 15th. At the time I was making around $600 a payday or a little over $1200 a month plus Cris' $75 child support payment. If you are living pay check to pay check and one pay check is plucked out of your hand you are in serious financial trouble. I didn't have any savings so financially I went in the hole for about two months. During that period, Dannielle and I went back to eating macaroni and cheese and lots of peanut butter sandwiches. Consequently, some of the bills didn't get paid on time and I was afraid the utilities would get shut off. It seemed like I was constantly taking two steps forward and one step back. I still hadn't clawed myself out of the poverty cycle just yet.

When it pours, it rains. Not long after I finally got the furnace repaired I received a certified letter from the IRS. I was being audited for tax years 1976, 1977, and 1978. In other words, the three years Cris and I had been divorced. As it turned out, he had claimed Dannielle as a dependent and so had I. Of course he lost that battle since all the support he was providing for his daughter was $75 a month. I don't know why he thought he could get away with that charade but he certainly tried. Needless to say he had some money to pay back to the IRS and wasn't happy. All these years I had barely heard from him but he managed to call me after the audit and began cussing me out for a minute before I hung up on him. I decided since I was back on active duty I would change

Dannielle over to my military dependent and eliminate all confusion with the IRS in the future. I had no desire to be put through another audit because of his greed and/or stupidity.

My active duty contract with the Navy came up for renewal and of course I jumped at the opportunity to remain on active duty. My yearly evaluations were superb and my military training was completed on time. In a few months, I would be eligible to take the test for E-5 and couldn't wait. That meant a promotion, more pay, and a little more responsibility. After I renewed my contract, I decided to schedule an appointment with OB/GYN at NAS Dallas and discuss having a tubal ligation performed. I knew I didn't want any more biological children after what I had been through the last six years. Giving birth to Dannielle almost killed me and I've been barely able to support the two of us since Cris and I separated. The OB/GYN doctor and I had a long discussion. He was reluctant to perform a tubal ligation on a single, 28 year female who might change her mind. We agreed to wait six months and if I still wanted the surgery to call and schedule it. Six months later I cleared a few days sick leave with my commanding officer and had the surgery. I have never regretted my decision. Under the circumstances it was the right decision even though Dannielle always wanted a little brother or sister. I had no intentions of remarrying and going through this hell again. I also felt that if you can't support the child or children you have (including college), why would you keep popping out kids like pop tarts from a toaster. That is irresponsible and unfair to the child or children you already have.

Along came Doyle . . .

Shortly after I had signed my contract with the Navy for another year on active duty at the Navy Recruiting Office in Dallas, I met Doyle my third and to date last husband. Doyle had been driven to Dallas by his recruiter in Wichita Falls for his physical and testing. We started talking during his breaks and exchanged phone numbers. Doyle was a blue collar worker, welder by trade, who was recently divorced and wanted something different in life. He was the typical Texan dressed cowboy complete with the straw hat. He was my age, had brown hair, green eyes, stood about 5'8", weighed around 150 lbs., and had the cutest dimples. Doyle was completely the opposite of Bill or Cris. Maybe that is why I was attracted to him. Plus, he was funny and I enjoyed being around him since he made me laugh. He started calling me on the phone several times at home after work and eventually he drove to Dallas and took Dannielle and me to dinner. Doyle and Dannielle seemed to hit it off after a couple of hours. Doyle told me he liked kids and had a son, Jason, the same age as Dannielle. He said his ex-wife had custody but he got him on holidays and six weeks during the summer. I appreciated the fact that he spent time with his son and missed not seeing him as much since their divorce. Cris couldn't have cared less since he sold us out for a new car!

Doyle enlisted in the Navy a short time later and was scheduled to leave for boot camp in San Diego when we decided to get married. Doyle and I went to a justice of the peace in Dallas and got married without meeting each others parents. I called mom a couple of days later after Doyle had shipped out to boot camp and told her the news. Since this was my third marriage and I was only 29, it wasn't any big deal. I guess everybody was starting to think I would be following in the footsteps of my mother. Honestly, I was beginning to think the same thing too. Doyle was completely opposite of the other two and besides, how many times can you be unlucky at love? The answer to that is as many times as the two of you screw it up. Sex with Doyle was good, not great, but it was nice to have a man touching me and wanting me again.

After boot camp, Doyle had orders for Millington Naval Air Station, Memphis, TN., for his Aviation Electrician (AE) "A" school and would remain at Millington as permanent party. After he completed his lengthy (4 months) "A" school, he would be assigned to the flight line to work on aircraft. All total, Doyle would be at Millington close to five years. The military makes every effort to keep married couples on active duty stationed together so while Doyle was at boot camp I started looking for a position in Memphis. I lucked out and found another TAR position at the Navy Recruiting Office in Memphis. I would be working in the actual recruiting section doing stats and ensuring the recruiters met their monthly goals. This sounded challenging particularly since recruiters that missed their monthly goals three months in a year were fired.

Since I was a reservist on active duty, the military reimbursed me for the move to Memphis. I packed a U-Haul with all of Dannielle and my worldly belongings and off we went. A friend drove the U-Haul and I followed behind in the car. Dannielle and I were on our way to Memphis and a new life. I gave the ratty trailer back to mom when I moved and she sold it for next to nothing a few months later. Dannielle and I found a fairly nice apartment in Memphis not far from the recruiting office and settled in. I wouldn't see much of Doyle until he completed boot camp and his "A" school. Dannielle started school that year. I decided she would be better off attending school on base since Doyle and I would be applying for base housing and moving on base eventually. Dannielle's first year in school wasn't good. I was constantly getting phone calls from her teacher regarding her bad behavior in the classroom. Her teacher said Dannielle would not stay seated and had begun hitting and biting her classmates. I chalked it up to the recent move to Memphis as well as my marriage to Doyle and decided to talk to her to resolve the problem. Unfortunately, talking didn't fix it because I kept getting calls from her teacher.

One afternoon I took off work early and went to Dannielle's school, stood outside her classroom, looked through the small glass window in the door and watched her for about 20 or 30 minutes. What I saw bewildered me. She was running around the classroom singing, punching a few kids that happened to be in her path, and not obeying the teacher who repeatedly asked her to take her seat. This was just ridiculous. I opened the door to the classroom, walked in and slipped up behind her. Dannielle turned around about then and saw me. I was still in my military uniform and for some reason the classroom got extremely quite when I walked in. I had motioned for the teacher not to say anything and she had complied. The look on Dannielle's face when she saw me was priceless. She knew she was in serious trouble and she had been caught red handed acting like a fool. I simply grabbed her by the arm, escorted her out of the classroom and signed her out of school early that day. The two of us drove home in silence. She knew she was getting a butt whipping. As soon as we got in the house she got three licks with a thin belt and I never got another call from her teacher that year or for several years. I'm sorry, but sometimes kids need more than just a good talking to. Dannielle had been acting out quite a bit lately. Before we left Dallas for Memphis, I took Dannielle with me shopping for us some new clothes and a few other items we needed for the move. I believe we were in either Sears or Montgomery Wards department store in the ladies department when Dannielle decided to start swinging from all the clothes racks like a chimp at the zoo. She would swing from one rack to another causing the racks to fall over. I repeatedly asked her to stop but there was no ending her bad behavior, so I decided to forget the rest of the shopping and check out. When we get to the check out line, Dannielle blurts out "my daddy's in prison". The clerk looked at me like I was total trash and probably wondered how I was going to pay for my items. I told the clerk that her father wasn't in prison and I had no idea why my daughter had said that. The clerk looked at me with that look that says "sure lady". I finished paying for my items and quickly left the store. Dannielle never could explain why she said that but I suspect it was because she was afraid Doyle would try to replace her real father. Also, she probably didn't know how to rationalize or understand why her father wasn't around anymore. I tried to explain to her that no one could ever replace her father and that he was in the Air Force stationed in California. I told Dannielle her father would come to visit her as soon as he could. Cris had stopped by the trailer a few months earlier for a short visit and to tell us he was on his way to his new duty station, San Bernardino, California. Dannielle missed her father but there was nothing I could do about it. He did not want the responsibility of a family. How do you explain that to a five year old? I tried not to bad mouth Cris to Dannielle but he wasn't much better than my own father. Kids need both parents in the home helping raise them but you can't make a biological father be a real father. It's just so easy for them to skip out and dump the full burden on the mother. I hope Dannielle realizes that Cris was not who she thought he was and did little of nothing to help raise her. He sold his family out for a new Chevy and thought a $75 child support check every month made up for his absence. Well, it didn't. Dannielle wouldn't see her father again until 1985.

In 1980, when my one year reserve contract was up, the Navy offered me a four year reserve active duty enlistment as an YN3 assigned to NAS Millington. This was possible only because I had gotten married. At this time, the military still did not allow single parents on active duty. I was assigned to the personnel office on base and processed incoming and outgoing military troops. I liked Memphis. It is a great city with lots of things to do and now I had someone to do them with. Doyle, Dannielle and I had become a family. The three of us took day trips and enjoyed the entertainment Memphis offered—such as Graceland and the Peabody Hotel. Doyle and I were able to see Jerry Lee Lewis perform one evening at one of the jazz clubs downtown during the annual jazz and rib feast. That first year of our marriage was great! I started taking night classes at Memphis State University and had two years of college under my belt. Quite honestly, I was just taking classes and really didn't think I would ever graduate. The Navy encouraged enlisted personnel to attend college and they paid for 90% of it if you were on active duty. When it came time for promotion, the Navy usually selected the enlisted personnel with some college education. The next promotion cycle I was selected to E-5 the first time up. A few months later, Doyle picked up E-4 and we were notified that we were selected to move into base housing. Life was good and getting better. That summer, Doyle's son Jason, flew up from Wichita Falls to spend a month. Jason and Dannielle hit it off and everybody hated to see him leave. Doyle and I took a few days leave and drove Jason home. I finally got to meet Doyle's parents. They were nice enough but weren't used to the military lifestyle and couldn't follow a lot of our conversation. His father, who had never been in the military, was a blue collar worker, an auto mechanic I believe and a part-time farmer. They had a modest four bedroom home, a small farm and a few farm animals. They were definitely country folks. We took some pictures of all of us while we were there. The one I saved and still have in the photo book is me sitting on Doyle's lap with Dannielle standing next to me. Doyle and I are in uniform because his mother wanted to see what the two of us looked like together in military uniform. The visit was only for a couple of days and Doyle hated to leave Jason but it was time to head back to Memphis and resume our daily routines. Later that year, Doyle and I filed court documents in Wichita Falls seeking full custody of Jason but the request was denied. Doyle took this pretty hard and we agreed to try again the following year but didn't.

On May 18, 1980, Mt. Saint Helens in Washington State erupted. This is important because I was in an airplane, a P3 Orion, on my way to Okinawa, Japan, and we didn't know if we could continue our flight or be ordered to return to Memphis. My commanding officer had selected me to go to Okinawa to process the drilling reservists arriving on their two week summer drill. He thought I was best suited for this temporary duty assignment (TAD) since I was a former drilling reservist. Since Mt. Saint Helens was erupting and we couldn't fly through the ash or over Russia, our plane was diverted to Alaska, therefore adding about four additional hours to the flight time. We had to land at Elmendorf Air Base in Anchorage for refueling and were on the ground about six hours. I'll never forget landing and seeing a small herd of moose on the runway just staring at the airplane. Why were there moose on the runway and why was it still dark at 7:00 a.m. local time? We got breakfast in the chow hall while the plane refueled and waited for the sun to come up. The sun never did come up. It was still dark when we took off around lunch and this was May. I don't know how anyone could live in the dark like that. My two weeks in Okinawa was an eye opener. I had never been out of the country except Guam, so this was quite an experience. Unfortunately, I was a female. I didn't know it at the time but females are considered secondary citizens in Japan. If I went off base, it was almost impossible to get anyone to assist me, even if I was in uniform. One evening I decided to walk off base and eat at a local restaurant but none of the waiters would recognize my presence. After about 45 minutes, another sailor (male) came over to my table and explained to me their custom and was kind enough to order my dinner for me. Other than the great souvenirs, I really didn't care for Japan at all and was glad when the assignment was over and I would be headed back to the United States where women weren't secondary citizens.

Shortly after my return from Japan, Doyle and I bought a quaint little three bedroom, one bath house in Millington not far from the base. We managed to assume a VA loan and didn't have to pay much down. On base housing was alright but owning your own home is much better. Both of us still had three years left on our current tour, so buying a house made sense. This was the year that cable came out, 911 went on the telephone, and computers were making their way into offices. The world was changing but at the time I didn't realize how much.

In late 1980, the Navy came out with a new program called the Enlisted Commissioning Program (ECP) and after discussing it with Doyle I decided to apply for it. To be eligible for the program, you had to have at least two years of college with a 2.0 GPA or higher and walk on water evaluations. This program required affiliation with the on campus ROTC unit and the recipient must complete their four year degree in two years. Once you graduated from college, you were sent to Officer Commissioning School (OCS) in Newport, Rhode Island for training for three or four months. If you were successful in completing OCS, you were commissioned as an Ensign in the United States Navy. It would take me at least two and a half years to complete the program if I was accepted and I was already nearly 30 years old. I knew OCS was going to be very difficult but I really wanted to be a commissioned officer and this was virtually my only chance. Going from enlisted to officer is a big jump. It's like moving from blue collar to board room. The increase in salary was astounding but so was the responsibility that went with it. I was accepted to the program and received orders to the ROTC Unit at the University of Mississippi and was scheduled to begin college in the spring of 1981. I had about six months to prepare myself for the transition.

Since we were busy moving into our new house and fixing it up, time flew by and before I knew it, it was time to go down to the University of Mississippi. The university is located in Oxford, Mississippi, about an hour and a half drive from Millington. I registered for classes, found a one bedroom apartment not far from campus, bought a few pieces of furniture, and checked in with the ROTC Unit. My goal was to graduate from college in June, therefore I needed to attend classes during the summer as well. Doyle and I had agreed that one of us would make the trip every weekend—either I would drive to Millington or he and Dannielle would make the trip down to Oxford. The weekends were to be our time together as a family. Unfortunately, it didn't work out that way. My course work usually kept me bogged down on the weekends and our family weekends dwindled down to once a month. It wasn't long before this marriage was on the rocks too! After the first year of me being in Oxford and Doyle in Millington, the romance was gone. I was trying to complete two years of college in one and a half years. That didn't leave much time for anything else. I needed to get to OCS in the summer and not the fall because the winters in Newport, Rhode Island are brutal and I couldn't see me marching and jogging in that type of weather. Also, I guess I just wanted to get this over with. I knew when I started this adventure it was going to be extremely difficult but I was determined to finish it. Doyle and I agreed to a legal separation during my third semester of college and he was kind enough to keep Dannielle with him in Millington until I graduated in June. I guess I had thought the third marriage would be the charm but it wasn't. It was just easier to say good bye.

I graduated from the University of Mississippi the middle of June 1982, with a Bachelor of Arts in Sociology and Criminology, and a GPA of 3.62. I never thought it would be possible for me to actually graduate from college, but I had. Now it was time for OCS. Before I left Mississippi, I filed for a divorce from Doyle. Another failed marriage. At this point, I realized that no marriage was going to work as long as I was in the military. It was just too many balls to juggle and my career would have to come before a husband. Men had always let me down so for now, no more men.

Once again I was a single parent in the military about to embark on a new phase of my career. Since Doyle and I were in the process of a divorce, I had to make arrangements for Dannielle's care while I was at OCS. I had no choice but to ask my mother to keep Dannielle while I was in training. Dannielle was being drug from pillar to post but it couldn't be avoided. I only hoped she would understand and adapt. I would owe the Navy four years once I completed OCS giving me a total of 11 years of active duty service in the military. Since I could retire after 20 years, I would be foolish not to stay another nine years but it wouldn't be easy as a single parent. After graduation from college, I took a couple of weeks leave before reporting to OCS in order to pack Dannielle and my things that were still in the house and drive Dannielle to moms' house in Texas. Doyle and I had sold the house in Millington and split the proceeds. At this point, we were just waiting for the divorce to become final. Since I had a small car at the time, it was necessary to load some of Dannielle's things on the top of the car. This was really stupid but I didn't think there was that much stuff. I should have rented a small U-Haul because about half of the stuff on top of the car blew off into the Mississippi River while we were crossing the bridge. One big gust of wind blew it into the river. The wind on that bridge was horrific and there were no shoulders to pull off on and no stopping allowed on the bridge. So all we could do was keep driving and watch all that stuff blow into the river. This upset Dannielle and she said "mom, there goes all my things!" I felt really bad but there was nothing I could do. After a short visit at moms', I said good bye to Dannielle and headed out to Rhode Island. I didn't want to go but I had to. Hopefully, the three and a half months would go quickly. I was scheduled to complete OCS in October and after a two week leave, report to my permanent duty station, the Pentagon in Washington, D.C.

Up to this point in my life, OCS was my hardest challenge. I was 31 years old, out of shape, a smoker, couldn't run, and didn't know how to swim. Actually, I was afraid of water. It was June 1982, and the weather in Newport was fantastic. I excelled academically but couldn't run the mile and a half in the required time nor could I pass the swimming requirements. Therefore, I was on remedial swimming and jogging for over two months. There never seemed to be enough time. Looking back, I would have to say OCS was a lot like prison. Once you checked in you couldn't leave, you didn't have access to your vehicle while there, you shared a small room with two other women, all activities were dictated, we all wore the same uniform, there was no free time for television or just hanging out, uniform and room checks were twice a day, no contraband was allowed in the rooms, meals were served in the chow hall at a designated time, and there were no visitors unless scheduled in advance. I guess the only difference between OCS and prison was I was called officer candidate instead of inmate. This place even had mandatory fun day on Saturdays. Every Saturday from 7 a.m. until 1 p.m. we were required to participate in five sports. I never saw anything fun about mandatory fun day. During the week, we had classes starting at 8 a.m. and continuing until 4 p.m. with an hour lunch break. Everywhere we went was in military formation. Jogging and swimming were scheduled first thing in the morning before breakfast and showers. The drill instructors enjoyed waking us up at 5 a.m. and taking us outside to run the mile and a half without letting us use the bathroom first. We got a bathroom break after our run. How sick is that? Swimming was the worst horror. We were required to jump off a nine foot board into ten feet of water in an Olympic size pool and then perform various tasks. These tasks consisted of treading water for 45 minutes, floating for 30 minutes, jumping in with your uniform on then taking your pants off while treading water and making flotation devices out of them, and jumping off the board wearing a Mae West life jacket which weighed a good ten pounds dry. We also had to swim underwater two lengths of the pool while the top of the water was on fire. Remember, I couldn't swim and was afraid of water. The first time I was required to jump off that board, I couldn't. The swim instructor told the girl behind me to push me in if I didn't jump by the count of three. I shut my eyes, held my nose, and just walked off the end of the board. I thought I was going to drown before I could get to the side of the pool. After months of remedial swimming classes, I finally passed the swim test. I have not been in a pool since. Now, for the mile and a half run. The only way I finished the run in the required time (10:20) was because one of the African American Marine drill sergeants chased me up the last quarter mile hill pretending to be the naked black man with a butcher knife from the movie "Dirty Harry". At the time of the final run I had open bleeding blisters on both of my feet. I tried to quit OCS after about two months but they would not let me. The wardroom full of high ranking officers told me to suck it up and complete the program or I would be converted back to E-5 and discharged from the Navy. There was no leaving OCS unless I graduated.

My divorce from Doyle was final in August and I received a copy of the papers during mail call. I mention this because during one of my liberties (I only had two), I attempted to rent a car using my American Express Card and the charge was denied. Actually, the clerk was instructed to confiscate my card and cut it up. I knew I didn't have any pending charges on it so I asked to talk to the American Express representative on the phone and found out that Doyle had charged an engagement ring on my card and the card was now 90 days past due. Since we were divorced, the ring obviously was not for me. The nerve of that Jerk! I managed to rent the car, keep my credit card and resolve the matter over the phone but I will never forget that moment when I found out the charge was $600 for an engagement ring. Doyle didn't waste any time moving on with his sex life. I had a brief sexual liaison at the university with a marine seven years my junior but Doyle and I were legally separated and the liaison ended on graduation day. How long had Doyle been seeing this woman? Apparently he had been having an affair for some time since the charge on my American Express card was 90 days past due. Geez, he couldn't even wait for the ink to dry on the divorce papers!

I called Dannielle three or four times while I was at OCS and received a few letters from her. I missed her but I had to finish this. Finally, it was time for graduation pictures and only three weeks until getting out of this hell hole. Since I rarely made it to scheduled meals and was definitely getting plenty of exercise, I had lost around 15 pounds. My photo turned out spectacular. That was one of the best photos I have ever taken. By the way, since I rarely had time to eat, I lived off of Kit Kats hidden in the ceiling tile in my room. We weren't allowed food in our rooms or lockers. It was called contraband, so we resorted to hiding candy and pop in the ceiling tiles in our rooms. That was the only way I kept from starving. The Navy trained me to be a ship driver while I was at OCS and our class took a tug boat out to sea for training twice a week the last two months of my training. This was quite comical since I was too short to reach the huge wooden steering wheel on the bridge and needed to stand on a milk crate. Every time the captain would yell "hard left rudder or hard right rudder" (left and right turns), the milk crate would slide out from under my feet leaving me dangling from that huge wheel. Needless to say, the captain cussed me numerous times. Thank goodness I was never assigned to a ship during my career because the milk crates would have been quite an embarrassment. I was commissioned as an unrestricted line officer, Ensign, in the regular Navy on October 1, 1982. As much as I disliked OCS, it instilled a lifelong sense of ethical values in me which I didn't have prior to this. All cadets were taught and forced to live by the creed "I will not lie, cheat, steal, or tolerate anyone who does". If only the rest of society could live by this creed. Graduation day I threw my service hat in the air, grabbed my suitcases, and hauled ass out of Newport, Rhode Island. Looking at that place in my rear view mirror gave me great pleasure because it was like getting released from prison. I couldn't drive fast enough. I was so glad to be finished with college and now OCS. Hopefully, there would be no more "no pot, no window" days but once again I was wrong.

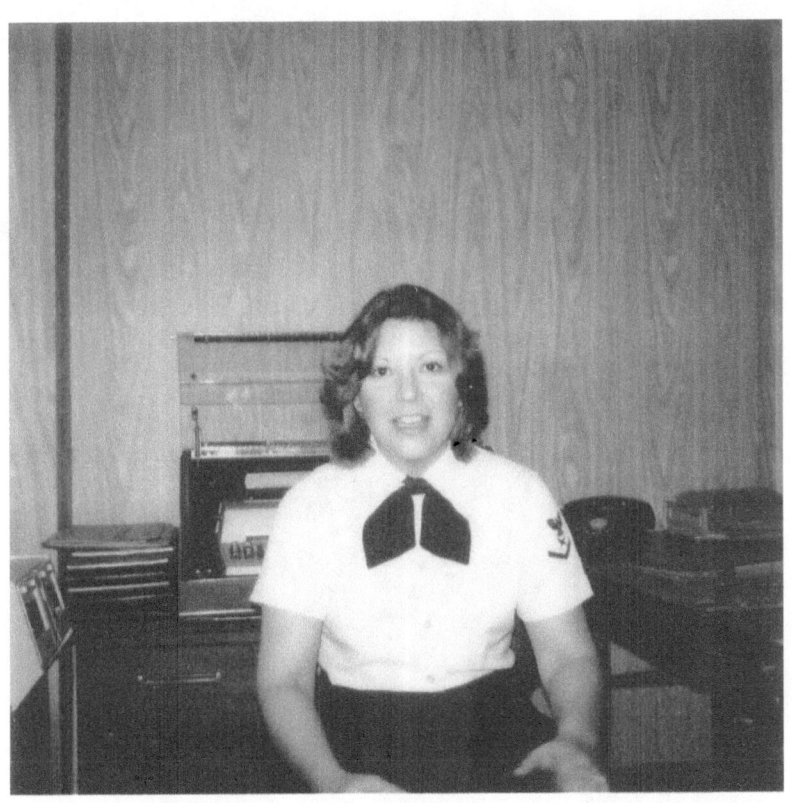

Me in my Navy uniform as a YN3, 1979

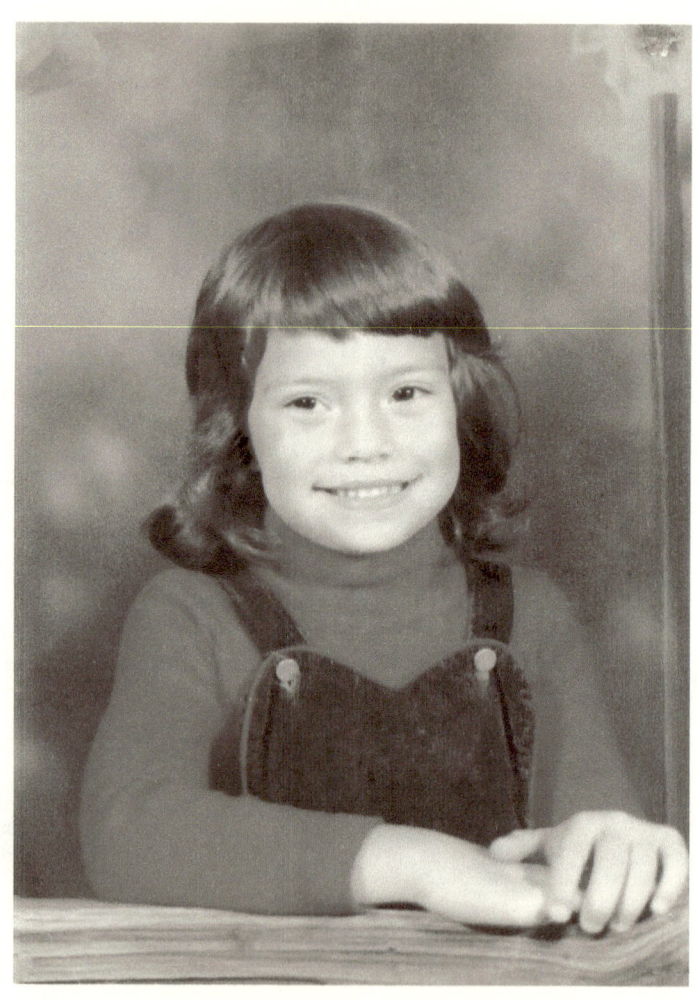

Dannielle, second grade photo, 1980

CHAPTER 8

Fighting And Surviving Breast Cancer (Age 32-37)

Fighting Breast Cancer Mentally and Physically . . .

During my two week leave, I found an apartment in Arlington, Virginia, bought a few pieces of new furniture I needed, scheduled the military movers to deliver my other belongings from Mississippi, and enrolled Dannielle in school. Since I didn't have time to drive to Texas, I arranged for Dannielle to fly from Dallas to D.C. The military always assigns a sponsor to new arriving personnel in order to expedite the transfer. Trust me, I needed it since the Washington, D.C. area is huge and I didn't know my way around. Driving in the metropolis is difficult if not impossible so most people, as I later found out, use public transportation. Thus, when I started working at the Pentagon it was a bus and a train every morning. The car usually stayed parked in the parking garage of the apartment complex. For me it was a new career in a new city and I was looking forward to reporting for duty at the Pentagon.

I settled into life in my new apartment and was adjusting to being a mom again as well as learning the ropes as a junior officer at the Pentagon. I was assigned to the Chief of Naval Operations, specifically the Fraud, Waste, and Abuse Program. The adjustment for Dannielle was more difficult than I had anticipated. I guess my absence over the last two years had left its mark. When she first arrived in Virginia, she told me several times she hated me and wanted to go live with her father. So one night when I had had enough, I packed her suitcase, told her to head out to California and I would call Cris and tell him she was on her way. Maybe that was mean but she never told me she wanted to go live with her father again. It took about six months for Dannielle to settle in

---

71

and adjust to the move to Washington. We had a great apartment with a pool, a new car, new furniture, new surroundings, and plenty of money for anything we wanted. It was a far cry from what we had three years ago—an old ratty trailer, a beat up orange Toyota with no heat or air, and living pay check to pay check. I was amazed and disappointed that Dannielle wasn't happy. I thought she understood that my absence had been necessary in order to ensure that she had a better life than I did. I guess it's hard for a nine year old to comprehend all of that. For me, life was good and I was certain that the struggle for survival was over. But I was wrong.

Being in the military on active duty, you soon make a circle of friends which become your extended family since your family normally doesn't live in the area. So was the case with me. At that time, I had two close friends, Mary and Charlita. I worked with both of them at the Pentagon and socialized with them occasionally after work. Mary was also a military officer a few years older than me, married to a civilian contractor, and they had a horse farm in Maryland not far from the Pentagon. Mary and her husband did not have any children and due to a medical condition, would never have biological children but they enjoyed having Dannielle up to visit and taught her how to ride a horse. Charlita was a civilian worker about my age, married to a Warrant Officer in the Navy, and they had two children about Dannielle's age. When I had to work late, Charlita would run and pick Dannielle up from school and watch her until I got home. I will always be indebted to these two women for the support they provided while I was a single parent at the Pentagon and even though I have lost touch with them over the last ten years, I will always consider them friends. There was one more friend I have to mention. Since living in the District of Columbia area is quite expensive and I had an extra bedroom, I decided to take on a roommate. Several people applied but I chose a young man, Gregg, who was right out of college and starting his career with the Secret Service. Gregg was just a nice guy with a mild mannered personality and we soon became good friends. Actually, it wasn't long before I started thinking of him as a little brother. Gregg and I were roommates for over three years. Dannielle and Gregg got along great and he didn't mind watching her at night occasionally. In the summer of 1983, I enrolled at George Washington University and started my masters' degree in Forensic Science. Gregg was kind enough to babysit Dannielle two nights a week until around eight p.m. while I went to school. I would drag home exhausted and the two of them would be sitting on the sofa watching television. I never worried about Dannielle when she was with Mary, Charlita, or Gregg.

While I was stationed at the Pentagon, I flew mom up from Texas for her birthday. She was only 59 but looked about ten years older and was in poor health. About five years earlier she had been diagnosed with type II diabetes primarily because she was roughly 75 pounds overweight and would not lose weight or change her diet. She continued to eat fried foods and tons of sweets therefore it was virtually impossible to control her sugar level even though she took insulin shots twice a day. Consequently, she also had high blood pressure, poor circulation in her legs and feet, poor eye sight, and a heart condition. My mother's health was rapidly declining and she was only 59 years old. Mom arrived with her one suitcase and her large cake Tupper Ware container full of prescriptions clutched in her hand. Since she had never been out of Texas (except Louisiana) or flown on an airplane, I was proud of her for making the long trip to visit. I tried to get her to move up to D.C. and live with Dannielle and me but she said she belonged in Texas and wanted to die in Texas. During mom's two week visit, the three of us did the usual tourist thing—we visited the monuments and the Smithsonian museums. The Viet Nam Memorial had just been completed and was open to the public so that is one of the first memorials we visited. It was so sad walking along that extremely long gray wall looking at the thousands of names of brave young soldiers who had lost their lives in a very unpopular war. I am a Viet Nam Era Veteran which means that I was on active duty military during the war but did not serve in combat. My knowledge of the Viet Nam War is primarily from textbooks, however most historians agree that this war was a black eye to the United States. A lot of our troops were treated badly after the war and they were generally not welcomed with open arms and parades when they returned home. Hopefully, history will not repeat itself. Mom was always exhausted by the time we got home but she was a real trooper and never complained. I really hated to see her leave but that was what she wanted. I think she felt overwhelmed by the size of the District of Columbia and wanted to go back to her little world in Texas. Coincidentally, today is her birthday. I'm typing this manuscript thinking about my mother and how nice it would be to call her and wish her happy birthday. Unfortunately, she passed away on May 13th, 2000, and I will never be able to tell her happy birthday again. Mother had been in and out of nursing homes since she was 55 but in 1993, she became a permanent residence at the nursing home in Athens, Texas. She died in that nursing home a pauper. Mom had spent her entire life looking for someone to take care of her and in the end she had no one, no assets, and no money. At the time of her death, she was confined to a wheelchair after having part of a toe amputated, was almost blind and was wearing adult diapers. She had allowed diabetes to take her life. Anne, Betty and I assumed she had life insurance but she didn't. Apparently, the policy had lapsed due to nonpayment while she was in the nursing home and she didn't tell anyone. I seriously doubt she was even aware that it had been cancelled since her diabetes had also caused dementia in her later years. Shame on me for not ensuring she had some type of will and life insurance policy at the time of her death. Mom had three children and we all failed her. My mother wasn't the best mother by any means but she was still my mother and I will always miss her. I wasn't able to attend her funeral and that will haunt me for the rest of my life.

Life for me changed forever in the fall of 1983 when I found a small lump in my right breast. I had just gotten promoted to Lieutenant Junior Grade and was having the time of my life. I went to sick call one morning to have it checked out and the doctor there referred me to the OB/GYN department at Bethesda Naval Hospital. It never occurred to me that I might have breast cancer since I was only 32. I even took a two week vacation to Hedonism II in Jamaica during this period and I'm glad I did because that is the last time I felt sexy and was able to wear a swimsuit without feeling self conscience about my appearance. I met a guy, Gary, the first day I was at the resort and we spent the entire two weeks together. Gary and I shared a bungalow and had wild, crazy, sweaty sex for two weeks. When we weren't having sex, we were doing tequila shots, swimming nude in the ocean, gorging at the buffet table or dancing by the pool. That two week vacation was the best vacation I have ever had. I was confident that the lump in my breast was nothing to worry about and didn't even think about it while I was in Jamaica.

In the '80's, breast cancer was still considered an old woman's disease. I was only 32 years old! The doctors at Bethesda initially treated the lump as a cyst and gave me antibiotics. I was on and off antibiotics for five or six months. The antibiotics were not doing any thing to shrink or get rid of the lump—it just kept getting bigger. The next thing the doctors tried was aspirating the lump. This meant sticking a needle into the lump and sucking the fluid out. Unfortunately, this didn't work either. After the aspiration, the lump got smaller but always came back within a couple of weeks. Eventually, the doctors at Bethesda told me they wanted to schedule a biopsy to determine if the lump, now determined to be a tumor, was benign or malignant. Since they felt confident the lump was a benign tumor, I wasn't worried. Well, it wasn't benign. The lump in my right breast, now the size of a golf ball, was determined to be a malignant tumor. I remember when the doctor told me I had breast cancer and needed a radical mastectomy as soon as possible. It was like someone had cut open my stomach and ripped out my guts. I screamed at the top of my lungs "no, not now"! I couldn't believe it. In 1984, breast cancer was pretty much a death sentence even with surgery and follow up chemotherapy and/or radiation. The follow up treatment was just too new and the five year survival rate was poor. I had just turned 33. Who dies of breast cancer at 33 years old? The doctors put a small drain tube in my right breast, scheduled me for surgery the following week, advised me to get my affairs in order, and sent me home. I called Anne when I got home from Bethesda to tell her the horrible news and she made arrangements to come up to be with me during surgery. After Anne arrived a few days later, I broke the news to Dannielle. I really don't think Dannielle understood that this was serious and

I might die. I believe I hand wrote a will since I didn't have one and gave it to Anne in case I didn't make it through surgery. About six weeks later, I had the legal department at the Pentagon prepare a legal will for me and discarded the handwritten one. The day of my mastectomy arrived and I was petrified. This was the first major surgery I had ever undergone. Thank goodness I had a very nice doctor, a young Lt. Commander, who helped me through this ordeal. And most important, I trusted him. Unfortunately I don't remember his name. Dannielle went to school as usual and Anne drove me to Bethesda Naval Hospital and stayed until I came out of the recovery room. The surgery took less than three hours. I remember going to sleep then waking up in the recovery room with my doctor calling my name. He told me to wake up that the surgery was over and he would be back later to talk to me about it but not to worry, everything was going to be fine. He also told me he had to remove part of my bicep muscle and my arm was in a sling but it was only temporary. That's all I remember until I woke up again a little later in my hospital room. Since I was an officer, I had a private room which was good and bad. By that I mean I wanted to be alone but I really shouldn't be because that's when depression sets in.

After I managed to come out of the anesthesia fog, I took an assessment of my physical condition and it wasn't good. I had a deep hole and stitches that were covered with gauze where my right breast used to be, two drain tubes coming out of my right side draining into a bag, my right arm was in a sling and I couldn't move it, and I had two IVs in my left arm. This was not good. What Mac truck had hit me? I started crying and couldn't stop. I really felt mutilated and wondered if I was going to survive breast cancer. Anne came into my room a few minutes later and tried to comfort me but it just didn't work. The doctors had me on morphine and other pain medications so I was in and out of sleep the rest of the day. The next thing I remember was being woke up the next morning by one of the attendants telling me breakfast had arrived. The attendant put the tray down and left the room. He didn't ask me if I needed help eating, he just left the room. I was starving but I couldn't move my right arm and there were too many IVs in my left arm to try to attempt to use it. How was I supposed to eat? I remember just sitting there looking at the scrambled eggs, bacon, toast, juice, pastry, coffee, and milk and wondering how I was going to eat and why no one cared. I really didn't need this insensitivity right now. I started crying and throwing a hysterical fit and rang the nurses' buzzer. When one of them answered and asked what I needed and I unloaded on them. I told the nurse that I couldn't use either of my arms and couldn't eat even though I was starving. The whole time I was crying and yelling about how insensitive they were. Apparently the nurses contacted my doctor because he was in my room a few minutes later. I was still crying so he calmed me down, apologized, and fed me my breakfast. While he was feeding me, he was discussing my prognosis. My physician said that he had removed 11 lymph nodes under my arm pits and two of the 11 were positive for cancer which classified my case as a Stage II. He also said I would need seven rounds of chemotherapy and possibly radiation therapy. Then he told me what I had been dreading hearing—even after chemotherapy, the chances of me surviving five years was about 70%. Five years is the time doctors have designated that is needed to consider the patient cured or the time required to determine if the cancer was going to rear its ugly head again. That's the horrible thing about cancer, if you've had it in one part of your body it very well may reappear in another location years later. I'll never forget how nice my surgeon was and how much time he took ensuring my hospital stay was a good one and my recovery progressed rapidly. For the next two or three days, he instructed an aid to assist me during meals and scheduled a physical therapist to come to my room several times a week to help me recover the use of my right arm. The biggest part of recovering from a major operation and/or illness is your mental state. If you stay positive and tell yourself that you are going to survive this, your chances of recovery are much greater. I knew I was going to recover from breast cancer but I also knew my life would be changed forever. No more taking life for granted and feeling invincible. And most importantly, I decided to live the rest of my life with no regrets. I wouldn't waste one single day of living because there might not be another. In thirty or forty years when I was old and gray and looked at myself in the mirror, I wanted to be happy with the reflection I saw. Thus, no regrets for the rest of my life however long that might be. I had a daughter to finish raising and I intended to do just that. I also decided she wouldn't have to go through all the hardships I went through because I would be there to help her with her life and help her choose the correct options. But first, I had to recover both mentally and physically. This operation had taken away my sexuality. I had no right breast, just a deep indention where it used to be. I felt like a butchered freak. The hospital psychotherapist counseled me several times before I left the hospital, but I never really got over the feeling that I was now a freak. I recovered the use of my right arm in about a week by doing wall exercises my physical therapist had shown me how to do. I stood against the wall and walked my fingers of my right arm up the wall going higher up the wall each time. My right arm was still weak, but at least I could eat by myself and wipe my butt without assistance. So many things you take for granted until you lose them, like the use of a limb. I was also able to shed the drain tubes and the two IVs in about a week and was up and walking around the hospital. Anne stayed about a week and a half and took care of Dannielle. I didn't want to scare Dannielle, so I asked Anne not to bring her to the hospital until I had the drain tubes out, the IVs out and the sling off my right arm. Dannielle was just ten years old and too young to see me like that. So after about a week, Anne brought Dannielle to the hospital to visit and it was really good to see her again. Mary and Charlita came to visit also. They helped me wash my hair and gave me a manicure which helped improve my self image. I was in the hospital close to two and a half weeks. Anne eventually had to leave, so Mary and Charlita took turns taking care of Dannielle until I was released from the hospital. I will forever be indebted to my sister as well as my friends for all the help they unselfishly provided during this period. Before I was discharged from the hospital, my doctor had a plastic surgeon stop by my room and talk to me about reconstructive surgery which could be performed after a year. The plastic surgeon said I had to complete chemotherapy and give my immune system time to recover from the treatment before he could start reconstructive surgery. In the meantime, I was given a mastectomy bra with a piece of foam in the right cup to wear. Dressed, I looked fine and almost got over feeling like a freak until I had to get undressed and look at my mutilated body. I had a nine inch scar running from my sternum bone all the way across my chest and under my right arm pit. Since it was necessary to remove my bicep muscle under my breast because the cancer had invaded it, my ribs stuck out and I could count every one of them. This is what I had to look at for the next year but I was alive. Cancer patients were assigned to the third floor at Bethesda along with Agent Orange patients. Agent Orange was a toxic agent used in the Viet Nam War to kill the foliage in the jungles in order for our troops to see the North Viet Nam soldiers. Unfortunately, it was later determined to cause cancer if inhaled which it was by many of our troops fighting in the jungles of Viet Nam. These Agent Orange patients weren't much older than me and were dying every day. That part of the third floor of Bethesda was the death floor. Death always seems to come in the middle of the night. Why is that? On two occasions, I was awakened around two or three in the morning by the sound of a woman wailing "no, don't go, don't leave me, please don't leave me". Then they would yell for their doctor and eventually a priest. Someone had lost their loved one. This was nerve wracking and it terrified me. I didn't sleep very well at night after the first incident and could not wait to get out of the hospital. Death seemed to be contagious on this floor of the Bethesda Naval Hospital. I know the doctors did everything they could to save those patients but sometimes it just isn't possible.

Since I wasn't scheduled to start my chemo for six weeks, I returned to work part time. The Navy calls it limited duty. I was only required to work four hours a day, was not required to perform extra duties or watches and my medical treatment took priority over everything else. Once I found out I had breast cancer, I took a six month leave of absence from my graduate program at George Washington University so the only thing I had to focus on right then was getting well. I started chemo in July, so Dannielle was out of school for the summer and went with me a couple of times. I was scheduled for seven months of the treatment receiving it by IV two times a month. In addition to the IVs,

I had to take a couple of prescriptions by mouth every day during this seven month period. Chemotherapy is basically a poison administered in a nonlethal dose which fights and kills cancer cells. My oncologist warned me of several side effects such as hair loss, weakness, nausea, vomiting, diarrhea, mouth sores and other immediate side effects of the drugs. He also said chemotherapy could cause early menopause and bone loss later in life. Well, he was right. I was sicker than a dog after every IV treatment but fortunately I never lost my hair. I did however lose most of my eyebrows so 15 years later I went to a permanent make up salon and had them tattooed back on. In addition, I started menopause at the age of 48 and have had both hips replaced but I'm still alive. Every time I went into Bethesda for my chemo, they drew six or seven tubes of blood for testing. Why they needed so much blood is beyond me but after being drained of that much blood and receiving chemo, I had absolutely no energy left. I would go home, take something for my nausea and go to bed the rest of the day. I'll never forget the taste that the chemo left in my mouth. It was sort of a disgusting metal taste, kind of like you had been sucking on coins or something. I never had an appetite during my two cycles of chemo every month. The thought of food turned my stomach so my doctor told me to take plenty of vitamins and drink lots of fluids. After several tests, it was determined that I did not need radiation therapy thank goodness and I looked forward to completing the scheduled chemotherapy. I couldn't move on with my life until I completed my chemotherapy and it was kicking my butt.

Since I was only allowed a six month leave of absence from my graduate program at George Washington, it was necessary to resume my classes about half way through my chemo. The school required a GPA average of 3.0 for all course work and I was worried I would no longer be mentally or physically capable of completing the program and meeting those requirements. Taking two classes a semester, I still had three semesters left which included one semester in the pathology department at Walter Reed Army Hospital. I knew finishing my graduate degree was going to be extremely difficult, but I had to do it. I graduated from George Washington University in February 1986, with a master's degree in Forensic Science. Hopefully, I would have the opportunity to use it.

With my education completed, it was time to start my reconstructive surgeries which would take nine months to a year to complete. Even though reconstructive surgery is technically considered plastic surgery, it is still surgery. My first operation took over 12 hours to complete. At this point, I didn't care how long it took because I was tired of the freakish cavity in my chest where my right breast used to be. During this first operation the doctors would perform a breast reduction on my left breast where it would match my new right one, a tummy tuck and then remove part of a muscle from my lower abdomen. The fat from the tummy tuck and the removed muscle from my abdomen would then be slid under my skin up to my right breast area, thereby replacing the lost bicep and fatty breast tissue. The doctors were hoping there was enough skin in the breast cavity to shape and cover the fat but if not, they would have to do a skin graft. They would also have to create a new belly button since that is the path the muscle and fat would travel to my right breast cavity. I know it sounds complicated, but basically the doctors would be replacing what they had removed during my mastectomy with muscle and fat from my stomach—no implants. This sounded great except this procedure was brand new in 1985 and none of the plastic surgeons had performed it yet. I was the first patient at Bethesda Naval Hospital to have this particular operation and that is one of the reasons it took 12 hours instead of the scheduled eight. There were also complications during the surgery. Unknown to all of us, I was allergic to the anesthesia they used. Consequently, I got the dry heaves on the operating table during the surgery. I knew something had gone wrong because I had an out of body experience during the operation. I remember being above the operating table, floating I guess, looking down at my body and watching the doctors perform the operation. I could also hear them talking to each other about me and the surgery. This out of body experience only lasted three or four seconds but I remembered it clear as day when I woke up in the recovery room. I asked the two surgeons what had happened and they explained that I was allergic to Secconal which caused me to develop dry heaves during surgery and consequently my electrolytes were now out of balance. They also said the surgery took 12 hours instead of the scheduled eight because of the complications. I told one of the doctors that I knew something had gone wrong because I had saw myself floating above the operating table. The look on his face when I told him that was haunting. He either thought I was nuts or he wasn't telling me everything. I will always wonder if my heart stopped beating for a few seconds. I guess I'll never know. I was in the hospital about a week after surgery but thankfully not on the third floor. Since a muscle had been removed from my abdomen, I couldn't stand up straight to walk. It took around two months for me to finally stop walking like a hunch back. I had 118 stitches and my recovery time from this surgery was close to three months. The plastic surgeons wanted to create a nipple for my new breast so I later had two additional minor surgeries for skin grafts. I have to admit, my new breast looks pretty good and I have had a couple of doctors compliment me on the results. I am extremely happy with the outcome but I still feel awkward when I'm wearing a swimsuit even though I'm probably the only one who knows I have a reconstructed breast.

About half way through my chemotherapy, I decided to send Dannielle to stay with my mother for a few months and then visit her father in California for a few weeks during that summer. Dannielle was supposed to be gone six months. While undergoing chemotherapy, I wasn't capable of taking care of myself much less Dannielle. Chemotherapy sucks all your energy out of you therefore you spend most of the time in bed. Cris had remarried but still lived in San Bernardino and was still on active duty in the Air Force. I had the legal department at the Pentagon draw up temporary legal guardianship documents which I mailed to mom and Cris prior to Dannielle's arrival. The documents stated I retained full custody of Dannielle and could rescind the guardianships whenever I deemed necessary. I talked to Dannielle once or twice a week while she was gone and she wasn't happy at my mother's house or Cris' but I needed a little time to complete my chemo and get back on my feet. At the end of the summer, I called Cris and told him I was making arrangements for Dannielle to fly back to D.C. He informed me that he had hired an attorney and Dannielle was going to stay in California with him. Cris was ignoring my wishes regarding the temporary guardianship and using his logic that he had possession of Dannielle and there was nothing I could do about it. Well, this forced me to hire an attorney who was totally useless and just wasted my time and money. After about three months of nonsense, I took matters into my own hands. I decided to book a flight to California, take a cab to Dannielle's school, show the principal my divorce papers giving me full custody, take Dannielle out of school, get in the waiting cab and the two of us fly back to D.C. All went well and Dannielle and I were home in Virginia before 5:00 p.m. eastern time. Only then did I call Cris to tell him I had Dannielle. Because of the time difference between California and D.C., it wasn't even time for Dannielle to be home from school when I called. Cris started telling me he was going to call the FBI and file charges against me, so I simply hung up the phone. I didn't have to put up with his crap anymore. That was the last time I talked to Cris. I hope there is an open fire pit in Hell next to my father with his name on it in huge neon letters. Dannielle told me a little later that Cris and his new wife were using drugs. Nothing would surprise me when it comes to that flaming asshole. It was great having Dannielle home with me again—I had missed her. I'm afraid if I hadn't been bold enough to fly to California and get her she might never have come home. Unfortunately, this period of time has been a riff between the two of us. She is 36 years old today and we have for the most part been estranged since she was 19. Dannielle told me a few years ago that she resented being sent to live with my mother (who she did not like) during this period and that we would probably never have a good relationship. She decided to adopt surrogate mothers several years ago, one of which is Anne. I deeply resent my daughter, who I as a single parent struggled to raise, thumb her nose at me. I recently decided that since she chooses to exclude me from her life during the remainder of mine, she need not benefit in any way from my death. Today, she is married to her second husband, George, and has three children—one from her first marriage and two from her second. George is

European and has been in the U.S. legally for about eleven years. They live in a neighboring city about ten miles from me but I rarely see them. I regret not being able to spend more time with Dannielle as well as my grandchildren but during the past 16 years I have repeatedly attempted to maintain a meaningful relationship with my daughter but have been rebuked over and over. As a result, I have developed a thick skin regarding our relationship and decided if this is what she wants, then this is what she gets. Having breast cancer at the age of 32 was just plain bad luck. I certainly didn't ask to be deathly ill for the better part of two years. Sending Dannielle away for a short period of time while I completed my chemotherapy and got back on feet physically was the right thing to do and I have no regrets. Being a single parent is not easy and sometimes you have to make tough choices. I only wish Dannielle was mature enough to think of my needs instead of her wants. Anyway, I was glad she was back home to help me during my recovery from my reconstructive surgeries, particularly the first one since it left me a hunch back for a while. I couldn't even bathe myself for a couple of weeks and tired easily. It was nice to get her homemade get well cards again—they cheered me up.

Surviving Breast Cancer Physically, Mentally and Financially . . .

In the summer of 1986, I learned that a medical board had voted to temporarily discharge me from active duty due to my breast cancer. This was a surprise since I had returned to full duty five or six months earlier and was satisfactorily performing all of my duties. My commanding officer had advised me a couple of months earlier that my case was being referred to a medical board but since I had returned to full duty I was confident the board would vote to retain me on active duty. I was wrong. I was discharged from active duty less than a month after the medical board had reached their decision. I would not be allowed to return to active duty for a minimum of three years and only then if I passed a military physical. My pay during this separation was a meager $1100 a month but at least I still health care coverage. Dannielle and I could not live on that income and I don't know anyone who could. It was poverty level pay and I had serious doubts about finding a job in the civilian sector under these conditions. Once again I was forced into the "no pot, no window" syndrome. I had no idea what I was going to do or how Dannielle and I were going to survive for the next three years or longer. I didn't need this stressful financial struggle again, not while I was still recovering from breast cancer. I had only been cancer free for two years so my lifelong battle had just begun.

When my discharge orders arrived, I packed our belongings and had the military put everything in storage. I didn't know where I would be living once I left D.C. Since I had saved a few thousand dollars, I thought it might be nice to take the long route home, via the Bahamas. I booked an Amtrak ticket from D.C. to Orlando, Florida and loaded my relatively new Honda Civic Wagon on it as well. Dannielle and I arrived in Orlando, waited for them to unload the car, and then took off for Miami to catch our cruise ship. The three day cruise was fantastic and Nassau was beautiful but now it was time to start driving to Texas. Since I didn't' have anywhere else to go, I called mom and asked if we could stay with her and Ray for a few months and she agreed. Dannielle and I moved into mom's garage apartment and I paid her rent every month. The garage apartment had two twin beds, a dining room table and chairs, a couple of dressers, a small desk with a television sitting on it, a kitchenette area, and lots of plants. It didn't have its own bath, but it was perfect for the two of us. After all, I only planned on staying there for a couple of months. I set up my portable IBM Selectric typewriter and started making my resume'. I planned on sending out a zillion of them, finding a job quickly, and moving out. Well, that didn't happen. As it turned out, no one was willing to take a chance and hire a recovering breast cancer patient. I don't know why but if I was talking to someone face to face and told them I was a recovering cancer patient, they backed away from me like I was a leper. I'll never forget thinking how ignorant these people were because cancer isn't contagious. My endless job search included the federal government, the post office, the local police departments, and even the city jail. I think part of the problem aside from my physical condition was the fact that I had an advanced degree and no practical experience in my chosen field of law enforcement. About the only experience I had was security guard training which I had undergone while in D.C. That was it. Not much to put on a resume'. My six months of unemployment benefits would run out soon and I had gone through most of my modest savings so it wouldn't be long before we were living pay check to pay check again. This was like a bad dream—1976 all over again. I decided to gain some experience in the law enforcement field and enrolled in the Texas Peace Officer Academy that fall. Dannielle started school about that time so my days were free to attend the academy. The academy was held in Athens and was four weeks long. It was nice to be out of the house and doing something again. I actually looked forward to getting up in the mornings. The academy was fun and taught me a lot about being a street cop which would come in handy a few years later.

About this time, mom started acting squirrely. By this I mean her diabetes was getting out of control and she was walking the house at night doing strange things such as pulling the pot plants out of their pots and eating them thinking they were turnip greens and going through my dresser drawers looking for dish towels she accused me of stealing. All of this was happening in the middle of the night and she did not remember any of it the next morning. I really didn't know what to think of all of this until I accidently discovered the remnants of her late night desert snacks under her bed when I was vacuuming her bedroom. There must have been 25 or 30 saucers and bowls pushed up under her bed that she didn't want any one to find. No wonder she was acting so nutty. Even though she was taking her insulin it wasn't doing any good because she was gorging herself on sweets sending her sugar level sky high. When I confronted her about it she became extremely agitated and told me it was her house and she could do whatever she wanted to do. After that spat, I stopped vacuuming her bedroom and didn't clean up the dishes under her bed again. I left mom alone about her eating habits because all it did was agitate her and I wasn't up for any more confrontations. We seemed to be getting on each others nerves lately, so I decided to ask Betty if we could move in with her and Tonya. Thanksgiving was in a couple of weeks so that seemed like a good time to make the move. Pete and Betty had recently split up, violently I might add. Both of them were having affairs and when they found out about each other's infidelities, a physical fight ensued. Pete threw Betty across the living room where she landed in the middle of the coffee table injuring her back and requiring hospitalization. After her recovery, Betty and Tonya moved out of the house and into an apartment in Gun Barrel City about 20 miles from Athens. Chris decided to stay with Pete which was a mistake because Pete was allowing him to drink beer and he was only 15 years old. A couple of years later, Chris was driving Pete's pick up truck intoxicated and not wearing a seat belt. Consequently, he ran off the road, hit a large tree, and was thrown from the vehicle landing on his head. He was in a coma for over a week and the doctors weren't sure he was going to live. Chris survived but was left with permanent brain damage. Today he lives in shelters and on the streets of Athens. This was such a tragic event that should have never happened. Chris was a great kid who wanted to be a veterinarian and I think he would have been a fabulous one. Tonya as it turned out was a crank head at the age of 13. Both of these kids had such potential. I blame Betty and Pete for these kids devastating outcome because somewhere along the way they quit being parents.

That Thanksgiving was a disaster. Mom and Ray had invited all the relatives over for the Thanksgiving meal that turned out to be horrible. At the time, mom drove a red Cadillac which was a tank but it accommodated her 300 lb. body. During one of her trips to town that week, she found a dead squirrel in the road and decided to bring it home to cook for Thanksgiving instead of turkey or ham. I couldn't believe it! I even offered to go to the store and pick up a ham but mom wouldn't have it. The road kill squirrel was green and smelled like hell. Who in their right mind serves road kill squirrel for Thanksgiving? Ray and I attempted to talk her out of cooking the road kill squirrel but there was no changing her mind. That thing stunk up the whole house while it was cooking. I didn't even look at it because I was afraid it had maggots in the pot with it. Along with the road kill varmint, she fixed macaroni and cheese and refused to drain the water off the macaroni thus it turned out to be soup and turnip greens which she had washed in the clothes washer with laundry soap. For desert she fixed a chocolate bunt cake which is the only thing anyone except mom ate that Thanksgiving. The ten or twelve guests avoided the stinky kitchen and did their best not to throw up. That was the worse meal I had ever had in my entire life. Mom couldn't understand why no one was eating her food with the exception of the bunt cake.

A couple of days after Thanksgiving, Dannielle and I had finished packing our belongings and were loading the car when a deputy sheriff showed up and said mom had called and asked them to send a deputy to escort us off her property. How insulting! I was paying her rent to stay there and cleaning her house yet she felt it necessary to call the police to have her daughter and granddaughter removed from the property. I can only hope this action was due to her diabetes possibly affecting her logic. It was several months before I talked to her again and that was only because Ray called and said she had gone into a diabetic coma and was in the hospital. Mom's health was going downhill quickly. She later apologized for calling the Sheriff's Department to escort us off her property and life moved on.

If I thought living with mom was bad, living with Betty and Tonya was ten times worse. My sister and inseparable childhood buddy was now a drunk and addicted to prescription narcotics. Tonya was a crank head, thief and juvenile delinquent. What happened to Betty and her family while I was gone? Is this the way I would have turned out if I hadn't joined the Air Force and left Texas? I think the answer to the last question is probably yes. I had my own problems dealing with breast cancer and unemployment but I knew it was only temporary. Betty's problems were permanent and this was sad. She got up in the morning around 7:00 a.m. and made a pot of coffee but instead of pouring herself a cup, she would fill the cup with whiskey and add two or three spoons of coffee to it. The first morning I saw her do this I just sat there at the kitchen table and watched. After downing this cup, she poured herself another and then another. All the time smoking cigarettes and not saying a word. Betty had drank three of her drinks in the time it took me to finish one cup of coffee. I was totally amazed. The worse part of this ordeal was she wasn't even tipsy. Then she would drag a few pills out of her purse and down them with her cup of whiskey. It took me a couple of weeks to figure out she was taking narcotics. After about 30 minutes, Betty would make her way to the bathroom and get dressed for work. She was currently working for her soon to be second husband, Bill, who was a wealthy attorney with a law office in Gun Barrel City. Apparently they had been having an affair for close to a year even though both were still married. Bill was currently awaiting finalization of his divorce and Betty had just filed for hers. To be exact, Bill, acting as Betty's attorney had just filed her petition for divorce. The prescription narcotics she was taking every day were samples she had stolen from Bill's brother who was a pediatrician and had an office next to Bill's law office. You can't tell me that someone didn't know Betty was stealing all those sample narcotics. They are controlled substances, so how was she getting them? I was never able to figure that out but a couple of years later, Bill's brother, the pediatrician, was convicted of illegally dispensing controlled substances and child molestation. Apparently, he was molesting some of his very young patients. He turned out to be a pervert. After Betty got dressed for work, she would pour herself another drink to take with her and finally ask where Tonya was. Tonya, who was now 14 years old, rarely came home at night these days and didn't attend school very frequently. Tragically, Betty didn't seem to care. Tonya had dropped out of school and was pregnant with her first of six children less than a year later. She had six kids before the age of 30 and I don't think any of them have the same father. While Dannielle and I were living with Betty and Tonya, Tonya stole a valuable dinner ring that mom had given me, pawned it and used the money for drugs. I confronted her, filed a police report, and started locking up my valuables thereafter. During the three months Dannielle and I lived with Betty and Tonya, Betty tried to kill herself twice. The first time by mixing alcohol and a hand full of prescription drugs and the second time by slicing her left wrist wide open with a butcher knife while standing at mom's kitchen sink. I saved her both times and she started calling me "miss goody two shoes". She also called me a bitch and said to quit interfering because she wanted to die. After Betty cut her wrist, the police asked me if I would commit her to the hospital for a mental evaluation and I agreed. She definitely needed help but I shouldn't have wasted my time because Bill, acting as her attorney, got her out of the hospital the next morning. Betty and Bill got married the next year and lived happily together until about seven or eight years ago. The two of them divorced but lived next door to each other on the lake in separate houses Bill had built. I heard the reason for their divorce was because of Chris and Tonya. Chris wouldn't take his medication and was subject to violent outbursts and Tonya stole them blind. Consequently, Bill did not want either of the kids in his house. I guess Betty felt responsible for them and refused to turn Chris and Tonya away. This riff with Chris and Tonya lead to their divorce and them living next door to each other in separate houses. I don't think they ever fell out of love and wanted to be near each other. Chris and Tonya were two beautiful children who had so much potential but their lives were ruined because of Pete and Betty's immoral lifestyle and their use/abuse of alcohol and drugs. Their two kids deserved so much more. I haven't seen Pete since 1987 but I considered him a farm animal. In 1976 when Cris and I separated and I went to live with mom, I thought it would be a nice change to have dinner with Pete and Betty and spend the night. Pete crawled in the bed with me in the middle of the night with a hard on. I don't know what he expected but I told him if he didn't get out of my bed immediately I was going to let out a blood curling scream, wake up the entire house and Betty could see him in my bed with his hard penis protruding from his boxers. He made up some excuse about drinking too much and left. I never told Betty what had happened but after that incident I kept my distance from Pete. What a waste of human flesh! If Pete is still alive today, he is probably married to some local drunken hag and still living in Athens. Bill died about three years ago from throat cancer and Betty is once again trying to kill herself. Last year she was in the hospital in a coma for five days as a result of alcohol poisoning. I am sure she will never stop trying to commit suicide and will eventually succeed. Betty and I are not close these days and haven't been since I lived with her and saw how messed up her life was and how powerless I was to help her. It's just sad—I was struggling to live and she was intent on dying. I couldn't take any more of the Texas crazies more commonly known as my family, so I decided it was time for Dannielle and me to go visit a friend (Dennis) in Memphis. I was proud to say I no longer fit in with the Texas crazies since I had matured, slowed down on my alcohol consumption, received a graduate degree, and wasn't interested in sleeping around. I wanted to visit Anne before I left Texas, so Dannielle and I drove to her house in Tyler to say goodbye. Anne had recently married her third husband, Ernie, who she had met at church. Ernie was divorced and owned a small appliance repair shop in Tyler. This marriage lasted twenty one years. As it turned out, Ernie wasn't the man Anne thought he was. He had skeletons in his closet. Fortunately, Mikelle and Paul were grown when they divorced. Since I was in Memphis and Spain during the majority of their marriage, I did not know Ernie very well but I'm sure the skeletons in his closet played a large role in their divorce.

It was such a relief to get out of Texas. I called Dennis and told him I was on my way and he didn't mind if we stayed with him for a little while. At this point, Dannielle and I were gypsies. Dennis was a former co-worker from my days at Millington Naval Air Station and we had stayed in touch over the last six years. He was a PN2 (E-5) on active duty in the Navy, originally from Little Rock, Arkansas, divorced with three children, and attending college part-time. Something I didn't know until 1987 was that Dennis was a closet homosexual and had a male lover living with him off and on. This explained why my sexual advances toward him never went anywhere. For years I had a crush on Dennis but he wasn't interested in me at all. While I was attending college at the University of Mississippi, I asked him down and we went to the Mardi Gras. While there, we slept on park benches together covered with newspapers for warmth and he never showed the least bit of sexual interest in me. Now I knew why. This was the spring of 1987 and before the "Don't Ask, Don't Tell" policy was enacted in the military, so Dennis had to be extremely careful who knew his secret. Wouldn't you know the one nice guy I had met in seven years was a homosexual? Just my luck!

I decided to apply to Memphis State and take a couple of post graduate classes while I was in Memphis. Since I was still trying to gain experience in my chosen career field of law enforcement, I took an Entomology class (study of bugs) as well as three semester hours in which I could write a thesis or perform an internship. I decided to perform an internship with the Violent Crimes Unit of the Memphis Police Department. My professor arranged the internship for me and I will always be in his debt because that summer provided me with experience I would probably never have obtained otherwise. This was going to be exciting. Not the Entomology class—it was boring—but the internship with the police department. I rode with the unit four nights a week, Thursday through Sunday, 11 p.m. to 7 a.m. This worked out great because Dannielle was asleep and Dennis agreed to stay with her at night while I was working. Before I started my post graduate classes, I needed to get my six month physical so I scheduled an appointment with the hospital at Millington. Thank goodness all was fine and I could continue with my plans.

During my two and a half month internship with the Violent Crimes Unit, my primary role was to determine cause and manner of death and assist with the processing of all crime scenes. In other words, perform the duties of a criminalist. The weather was warm so the crime rate was on the rise. The majority of violent crimes in Memphis occurred at night and usually in the projects. People kill other people for little or no reason, particularly if drugs and alcohol are thrown in the mix. Due to the risk of infection from HIV/AIDS, it was necessary for us to wear double gloves and covers for our shoes. We also were required to use triple body bags when transporting victims to the morgue. I think a chicken leg was the worse example of a needless death that I witnessed during my internship. Numerous residents of one of the projects were cooking out and drinking when the party got out of control. Apparently a fight broke out over who was going to get the last chicken leg and one of the residents pulled out a .22 and shot the man holding the chicken leg. When our unit arrived at the scene, the victim was deceased and the suspect was hiding in one of the apartments in the project. We secured the crime scene and processed it while the K-9 unit flushed out the suspect who was arrested and hauled off to jail. I'll never forget thinking how ridiculous this homicide was—a man died over a chicken leg. Another case I remember was a man shot his wife of many years in the left part of her chest with a shotgun because she insisted on saving part of their welfare check for groceries. The husband wanted all the money so he could buy his beer. The wad and lead from the buckshot had pinned the woman to the wall and the blast had lifted her about three inches off the ground. When our unit arrived on the scene, we saw this middle aged woman dangling from the wall with most of her left breast tissue imbedded in the drywall. The husband had shot his wife from a distance of approximately five feet with his shotgun in her left breast because that is where she put the $32 she had saved from their welfare check. I dug the woman's breast tissue, along with the bloody $32, out of the wall with a pocket knife and processed the victim for transport to the morgue. The police officers at the scene took the husband into custody for homicide and all the time I'm thinking what a waste. This drunken asshole killed his poor wife in this horrific manner because she wanted to save $32 of their welfare check for groceries. I hope he got life in prison for this. This was the way the summer went—one dead body after another. Our unit processed four to six scenes a night. We processed a couple of scenes off of Interstate 40 where motorists had discovered two young women who had been sexually assaulted and strangled then dumped like trash on the side of the road. Our unit was afraid we might have a serial killer. As it turned out, we did and the case was investigated by the homicide department. Later in the summer, we were called to a house of an elderly man who had no air conditioning and subsequently succumbed to the heat in his house. He was afraid to open the windows, so he just sat in his recliner until he died from the heat. Actually he sat there and cooked in his recliner. The neighbors complained of a foul odor coming from his home, so our unit was called. By the time we discovered his body, he was in deep decomposition and we had to scrape his body fat and tissue off the recliner in order to remove it for transport to the morgue. The temperature in that house was well over a hundred degrees and the smell was horrendous. The poor man even had maggot infestation in his mouth and eyes. That was a really pathetic, disgusting crime scene to process. It was determined that the poor old man died from natural causes but he shouldn't have. He died only because no one bothered to check on him for over a week and only then because the smell had become overpowering. Where were his friends and relatives? I could go on for pages revealing the cases our unit worked that summer, but I think you get the idea of how my summer went. I gained invaluable experience working with the Violent Crime Scene Unit in Memphis but I wasn't sure I was capable of doing this work day after day for the next ten or twenty years. It makes you cynical because you see the worst of mankind and start to wonder where all these animals come from. Did they fall from the sky in the middle of the night and no one noticed? What had happened to our society over the last twenty odd years? I guess we had created these monsters and there was no putting the genie back in the bottle. I completed the Entomology class and my internship, thanked Dennis for his kindness and hospitality and packed the car once again. The summer was ending and it was time to enroll Dannielle in school somewhere, so I thought we would head down to Florida for awhile, maybe Jacksonville.

Since I had a little time to kill, I decided we would drive down to the Keys, stop at Tampa, and then settle in Jacksonville. I didn't have much money so I bought a mosquito net and a full size air mattress to put in the back of the Civic for us to sleep on. Dannielle and I toured Florida during the day and stayed at KOAs at night. It was perfect since the campgrounds had a pool, a kitchen, a full bath, and they only cost $12 a night. Eventually it was time to look for a one bedroom apartment in Jacksonville. A one bedroom was all I could afford so Dannielle and I would have to share the bedroom. I was lucky enough to find a nice apartment less than a block from Dannielle's new school and in a fairly nice neighborhood. Since we didn't have any furniture, it didn't take us long to unpack our clothes, a small television and a boom box I had in the car. I bought another air mattress, a card table and two fold up chairs for the kitchen, rented a sofa, and got some milk crates to use as nightstands and dressers. The apartment was now furnished. This is the way Dannielle and I lived for five or six months. She went to school during the day and I dealt with my creditors and looked for a job. At least now I had some practical experience to add to my resume'. After a couple of months, I decided to send my resume' to the Texas Board of Pardons and Parole and apply for a parole officer position. My degree in sociology and my Texas Peace Officer's License helped me get the job. After performing a through background investigation on me, I was notified by mail and telephone that I was hired as a state parole officer and would be based in Sherman, Texas. I would be required to attend a two week training class prior to assuming my duties, but I could start work in about a month. Finally, a job! I had just completed my six month physical check up at Jacksonville Naval Hospital and was still cancer free. I had been cancer free for over three years now and unemployed for 15 or 16 months. I was definitely ready to go back to work. I was tired of being a broke gypsy.

It was early 1988, when Dannielle and I arrived in Sherman, Texas. Sherman is relatively small town located north of Denton and only about 25 miles from the Oklahoma state line. Before I took this job, I had never heard of Sherman, Texas. I found a small two bedroom apartment for us to live in, bought some used furniture, and enrolled Dannielle in school all in one week. Life was getting back to normal for Dannielle and me. We had real furniture again instead of air mattresses and milk crates and I was drawing a paycheck. We could actually afford things like food and new clothes. Being poor sucked! I hoped I would never again experience the "no pot, no window" plight.

Being a parole officer takes a special type of person because you are part social worker and part police officer. At the time, Texas did not allow parole officers to carry firearms even though they were considered law enforcement officials and cell phones were not yet invented so all I had was my badge and a 14" Maglight flashlight that I kept on the front seat. The year I started working as a parole officer, five Texas officers had been murdered by parolees. This is a stressful, never ending, and dangerous job. My caseload ranged from 90 to 110 parolees and I took case files home at night just to stay caught up. By state law, parole officers have to make a certain number of contacts each month with a parolee they are supervising. The number of contacts is determined by the type of crime they committed and the risk to society they pose. Usually a parole officer will see the parolee twice a month in the office, once a month at home, and every month or every other month at their place of employment. Parolees are required to have a permanent residence prior to being released from prison and be actively seeking a job once they are released. Eventually, employment is a must for every parolee. Strict supervision of parolees is necessary in order to protect society and hopefully prevent the parolee from reoffending. Unfortunately, even with the best of supervision statistics show that about 75% of parolees will reoffend and be sent back to prison. A lot of the parolees become institutionalized and prefer prison life so they reoffend soon after they are paroled in order to return to prison where they feel more comfortable. Others, on the other hand, sometimes chose to violate their parole and run soon after their release. Since Sherman was so close to the Oklahoma border, several of my parolees violated their parole and moved to Oklahoma without permission. About once a month I was faxing my warrant to the Sheriff's Department in the Oklahoma county right across the state line and asking them to pick up the absconded parolee. Unfortunately, once the parolee was in their custody I had to drive to Oklahoma in my personal vehicle, pick up the parolee at the jail, and then transport him or her to the jail in Sherman. I would handcuff the parolee to the door handle in the back and the parolee and I would return to Sherman. If I remember correctly, we only had 72 hours to pick up a parolee from Oklahoma or the Sheriff's Department had the option of releasing them and they usually did because they did not have the funds or space to house an absconder indefinitely. Me transporting absconders in my personal vehicle was very dangerous and I didn't particularly like doing it. If one of my parolees reoffended or violated their parole I was required to obtain a parole warrant for their arrest and with the assistance of the local police department arrest the parolee and take him or her to jail. Being a parole officer made me street smart. I learned all the prison and gang tattoos and most of the con games. These things aren't taught in college. After a few months on the job, I decided to join the Sherman Police Department as a reserve police officer. One weekend a month I patrolled the streets of Sherman with a veteran police officer. I got to know all the officers fairly well and when I needed assistance arresting a parolee they were always there to help. In other words, they had my back. I depended on their help since by law I couldn't carry a weapon while performing my duties as a parole officer.

The Parole Office in Sherman only had a total of three parole officers and the area was primarily rural, therefore I spent a lot of time driving out to the sticks by myself making home visits and verifying addresses. This, coupled with my frequent trips to Oklahoma, prompted me to seek a position at another office. I had been at the Sherman office about ten months when I was notified that there was a Parole Officer position now available at the Tyler office and of course I took it. Dannielle and I once again packed our belongings in a U-Haul truck and moved to Tyler. On this move, I decided to have the military deliver my household belongs out of storage because I was tired of living with little or no furniture. There were seven or eight parole officers assigned at the Tyler office and the parolees for the most part lived in the city. Hence, my caseload was a little lighter and I didn't spend so much time in the car looking for addresses in the sticks. Additionally, the Tyler office had a drug and alcohol testing unit which Sherman did not. I liked my job again. Dannielle and I settled into our new apartment and life was good. I was busy at work, Dannielle was enjoying school, and time flew by. I had all but forgotten about the Navy and the possibility of returning to active duty until I received a letter from them in the summer of 1989. The letter stated that if I passed a physical exam, I would be eligible to return to active duty at the rank discharged and I could choose my next duty assignment. I couldn't believe it! Of course I wanted to return to active duty and hopefully retire in five or six years. I called the number provided on the letter, accepted their offer and asked for a European tour with Naval Criminal Investigative Service (NCIS). The lady on the other end of the phone line simply said "OK". It was that simple. She offered me two or three options for duty assignments but I accepted a three year tour at Rota, Spain. This tour could be extended one year but that decision was based on the needs of the Navy. Dannielle and I were going to Europe! SWEET!

I scheduled a physical exam at NAS Dallas and I passed it with flying colors. This was a huge milestone because I had now been cancer free for over five years. The physicians considered me cured. The Grim Reaper could quit tapping me on the shoulder because I wasn't going with him just yet. Twenty six years later and there still is no cure for breast cancer. The detection and treatment have improved immensely but there is still no cure. Why not? All these years I've lived with the fear of it popping up somewhere else in my body. How much longer is it going to take to wipe out this deadly virus? I'm one of the lucky ones—I survived. Now I felt I could move forward with my life and accomplish anything so look out Rota, here I come.

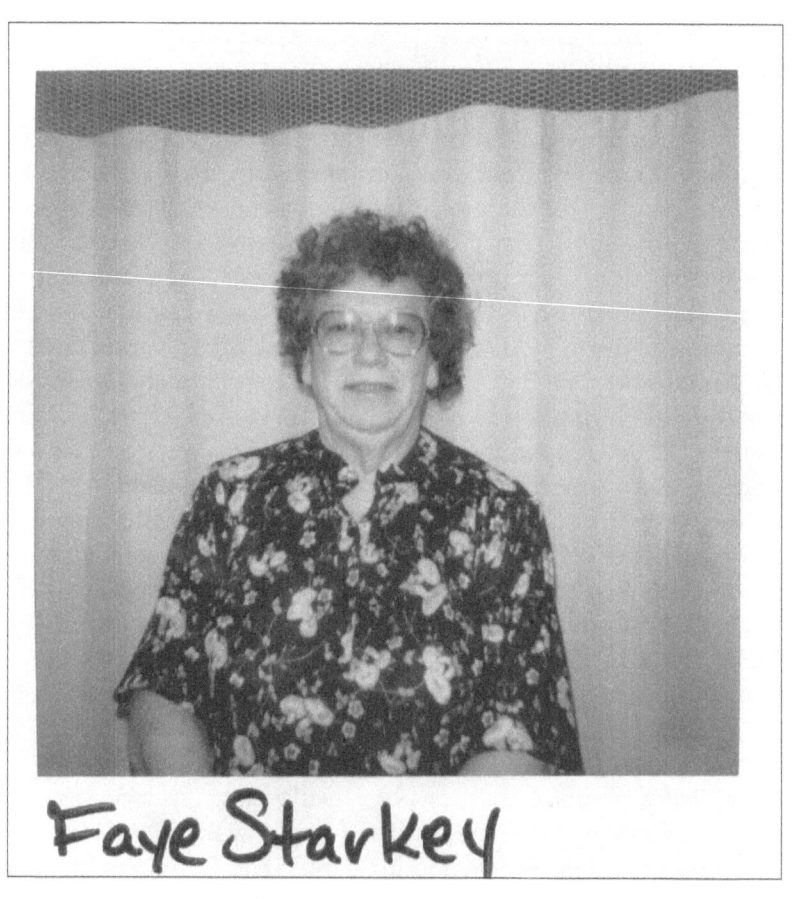

Faye Starkey

My mother, 1994, at the nursing home in Athens, TX

CHAPTER 9

NCIS And Military Retirement (Age 38-42)

Dannielle and I arrived in Rota, Spain on the last day of November 1989. Spain is really beautiful and the weather is always perfect. The average temperature is in the mid 80s with low humidity. Spain always has the most gorgeous clear blue skies. It very seldom rains in Spain, so the song was right—it never rains in Spain. Rota is a small city located on the southern tip of Spain. You can stand on the beach and look across the ocean and see northern Africa, specifically Morocco. How fantastic! It was a great day to be alive. I was the officer agent assigned to the NCIS office in Rota and as far as I knew, the only officer agent in that part of Europe. The uniform of the day was a suit like the civilian agents wore instead of my military uniform in order to prevent my rank from interfering with an investigation. Being a federal agent, you were never expected to get very dirty any way. This was my prize tour and most probably my last tour in the Navy before I retired.

After a very long flight from Dallas, Dannielle and I were met at the Rota Airport by one of the NCIS agents, Special Agent (SA) Milt. He drove us to the officer quarters on base where we lived for about a month while I looked for a permanent residence and waited for our household goods and car to arrive via boat. Over the next few days, I was busy checking into the base and enrolling Dannielle in the Department of Defense high school located on base. It was hard to believe Dannielle was 16 years old and was almost grown. It had been such a struggle to survive over the last 13 years I had lost track of time. Now I felt my financial struggle was finally over or at least I could see the light at the end of the tunnel. I was really hoping Dannielle would like her new school and enjoy being in Spain. This was a fantastic opportunity for both of us.

With the help of the other agents in the office, I managed to find a very nice gated three bedroom, two bath house with a pool in the Spanish community not far from the base. It wasn't long before our household goods and car arrived and Dannielle and I began settling in to our new home and our new life. At that time, the houses in Spain didn't have central air or heat probably because of the cost involved and the almost perfect weather. During my stay, the coldest I remember it getting was 45 degrees and the hottest, around 90 degrees. In order to keep the houses cool in the summer, the floors were tile and the windows were shutter type without screens that opened up wide to let the breeze blow through the house. Therefore, we bought and used fans and heaters which kept us comfortable. Besides, if it got too hot Dannielle and I could always go jump in our pool. I loved our pool but I hated cleaning it every day. The winters only lasted around three months so the pool was in use the majority of the year. During the peak of summer, it didn't get dark until after 11:00 at night so if you were so inclined, you could stay in the pool until the wee hours of the morning. In order to cook on the stove or have hot water to shower and wash the dishes, it was necessary to buy bottles of Butano which are similar to Propane here in the U.S. It was a must to always have at least three bottles of Butano on hand. It very seldom rained in southern Spain and never snowed but once or twice a year the African winds would blow through and there was orange dust everywhere. The best thing to do during these dust storms was just stay inside because you couldn't see two feet in front of you and it was very difficult to breathe. Dannielle and I loved the Spanish culture. The people were extremely friendly and there was no rat race. Every day they observed siesta in the afternoon from one to three o'clock. All the shops, banks and government offices shut down during this period of time for their traditional siesta. This was the little block of time the Spanish set aside during the day to rest. I really wish this custom would be adopted in the states. There were no malls, large parking lots, or traffic jams in Rota. Their culture was focused on the family and enjoying life. I loved the Spanish lifestyle because it was so peaceful and seemed to be a better way of life. The downtown streets were too small to accommodate vehicles since they were built many years ago for pedestrians and bicycles so most people just walked and left their vehicle at home. I shipped two televisions to Spain but since there weren't any English channels except the Navy news, Dannielle and I usually rented VHS movies from the video store on base. Our home had a telephone but it was expensive and sometimes difficult to make overseas phone calls so it was primarily used for emergencies only. I did try to stay in touch with mom and called home every four or five months but it was easier to just drop a letter to her in the mail. Remember, this was 1990 and before the big technology boom so snail mail was still prevalent. Mom's health was declining rapidly but thank goodness Ray was there to help her. Since I didn't speak Spanish, I was required by the Navy to attend one hour Spanish classes five days a week during lunch for about six months. Dannielle was taking Spanish in school and it wasn't long before both of us became relatively fluent in the language. This was really essential since we lived in the Spanish community and I would need to know the language in order to converse with the Spanish police during the investigation of some of my assigned cases.

I wasn't allowed to work cases until I attended a five week training school at the Federal Law Enforcement Training Center (FLETC) in Glynco, Georgia, so for the first three months I performed background investigations on Navy contract personnel desiring employment on the base. When I was finally able to attend training at Glynco, Dannielle stayed with one of the agents, Ruben, and his wife. Ruben and his wife didn't have children and they insisted Dannielle stay with them in my absence. I think this was a real learning experience for them since Dannielle was 16 years old and not a small child. Teenagers are sometimes difficult to understand much less get along with and Dannielle was no exception. I graduated from the training academy and Ruben, his wife and Dannielle managed just fine in my absence. You just have to have a lot of patience with a teenager.

After I returned from FLETC, I started working an array of cases assigned to me by the Special Agent in Charge (SAC), Dan. NCIS only works felony cases involving Navy personnel and/or their dependents regardless if the incident happened on or off base. My caseload consisted of rapes, sexual assaults, death investigations, theft, fraud, black marketing, and a couple of drug investigations which I was the assisting agent. In 1990, DNA analysis was just emerging on the scene as an investigative tool but was not yet accepted in courts. Therefore, we worked cases the old fashioned way—fingerprints, crime scene photos and sketches, interviews, and collection of physical evidence. Most of these techniques seem antiquated today since forensic science technology has made leaps and bounds over the last 15 years. I also attended several autopsies and soon learned to put Vicks up both my nostrils to combat the smell. One of my cases involving theft and fraud allegations against a Lt. Commander (LCDR), one rank above me, resulted in a court-martial which was a new experience for me. A court-martial is the military equivalent of a trail in the civilian sector. This case was difficult to investigate and very time consuming since I had to testify at the court-martial but in the end he was convicted by a jury of his peers of theft and fraud and sentenced to Fort Leavenworth Prison for five years. I still have the Navy Times newspaper article showing the LCDR being taken out of the court room in handcuffs. The crime rate in Rota was low but I was kept busy and the months flew by. My solvability rate was 65% which was slightly above average so I felt I was living up to NCIS expectations. This was important to me since I was the only officer agent assigned to Rota. I didn't want the other agents to think I was a slacker and couldn't perform my duties. I always felt like I had to be as good as or better than the civilian agents. Additionally, after a little practice, I excelled on the firing range. I hadn't fired a handgun or shotgun since my training to obtain my Texas Peace Officer's license in 1986, but it all came back to me. The only thing I didn't excel at was running the required mile and a half every six months. I always passed it but just barely. I hated running and that never changed. I would have rather taken a beating than run that mile and a half. I always thought the Navy would have been wiser to extend the time limits slightly and require a very fast walk instead of a run since pounding that pavement caused many injuries and played havoc on your knee and hip joints.

In the summer of 1991, not long after Desert Storm, I decided to take some leave time, bought a Euro Rail ticket, and Dannielle and I traveled around Spain, Germany, Italy, France, and England for about two and a half weeks. This ticket allowed you to get on and off the train whenever and wherever you wanted so we were able to make many stops and see so many historical places in Europe. We either slept on the train or stayed at hostiles thus keeping the cost down but still having a marvelous time. We went to Madrid, Barcelona, East and West Berlin, Munich, the French Riviera, Paris, London, Milan, Rome, Venice, and Nice. Anywhere we decided to get off the train we did. This was simply a marvelous vacation which we would never have had the opportunity to experience if I wasn't stationed in Rota. The places I enjoyed most during this vacation were London and West Berlin. Dannielle and I went to the Tower of London and the museum at the tower and did some shopping at the famous department stores located in downtown London. We stayed at a quaint hostel in West Berlin for three days and enjoyed it immensely. The Berlin Wall had just been torn down so we were able to collect some of the rocks from the wall for souvenirs. West Berlin was very commercialized sort of like a mini Las Vegas but East Berlin still reeked of communism. We only spent a few hours in East Berlin because the depressed economy and the cameras on every street corner gave me the creeps. Another city I did not enjoy during this vacation was Paris because the locals did not seem to like Westerners and were not very hospitable. I had planned on staying two days there but left after only one night in a hotel. Dannielle didn't particularly care for Venice because it is a floating island and she was sea sick the entire two days we were there. I kept thinking she would eventually recover enough to go sightseeing with me but she never did and subsequently spent most of the time in our hotel room in bed. We collected many souvenirs from out travels and took lots of pictures for keepsakes. On the way home, we stopped in Sevilla (Spain) to attend the Expo being held there that summer. I don't know what I expected an Expo to be like, but it wasn't that enjoyable to me because of the thousands of people and the constant walking.

Before Dannielle and I knew it, our European vacation was over and it was back to our normal routine in Rota. A little later that summer, Dannielle was fortunate enough to get a ticket to the Madonna concert in Madrid. A few of her friends went with her on the train to the concert and she had a fantastic time. Also that summer, we decided to attend a bull fight in Rota with some of the other agents. This was another once in a life time experience but one I wished I had skipped. I didn't consider it much of a fight but more of a bull slaughter because after being stabbed in the neck ten or twelve times by the matador, there was no way that bull was coming out of the ring alive. After the fight and the bull was dead, he was hung up by his feet and his meat was sold before the next bull fight started. Dannielle and I stayed for two fights and left. I just couldn't get into that Spanish tradition. We also took a one day bus tour to Gibraltar which is a tiny section of Spain still owned by the British. It is the home of British Petroleum (BP) but inhabited primarily by migrated Indians. There wasn't a lot to see or do there but I'm glad Dannielle and I were able to visit the rock of Gibraltar.

The second year of my tour, our villa was broken into twice within a matter of about six months. Both times were by means of our shutter windows and both suspects were male heroin addicts on furlough from the Spanish prison. Heroin addiction is prevalent in Spain therefore there are a lot of heroin addicts in prison. The Spanish prisons are different than the ones here. The family of the inmate is responsible for the inmate's care and must provide food, clothes, and medical attention. The prison only houses the inmates and they are allowed out of prison twice a year on furloughs to visit their families. These addicts are ordered to remain at home during their furlough but they always seemed to slip away in search of another fix. I guess our house looked like a good mark since it was expensive, hidden by a wooden fence and trees, and no one was usually home during the day. The first break in occurred a few days before Christmas and the jerk actually opened most of the gifts under our tree and picked out what he wanted or I should say what he thought he could pawn for drugs. He even had the audacity to fix himself a meal in the kitchen. The second break in happened a few months later while Dannielle and I were outside watering the plants. Dannielle went into the house to use the bathroom and found the perp in my bedroom going through my jewelry box. He saw her, jumped out the bedroom window and ran around to the front of the house where I tackled him. I had heard Dannielle screaming but I couldn't understand what she was saying. I figured it out when I saw the shabby looking man run from the back of the house toward the road. After I tackled him and had him on the ground sitting on him with his arms pinned behind his back, I asked Dannielle to go in the house, get my handcuffs and call the Spanish police. The nerve of this ass! The Spanish police arrived a few minutes later and frisked him. That is when we found the switchblade knife hidden in his left boot. I'm glad I never took my hands off of him after I handcuffed him because he could have very easily bent down and grabbed the knife. Even though I was a special agent, the Spanish government didn't allow any of us to carry our weapons off base. Fortunately, I knew the majority of the National Police and the La Guardia Civil and when the call came in from Dannielle saying we had an intruder, they responded quickly. After this second break in, I decided to move into town where we wouldn't have to worry as much about another addict looking for an easy mark. The following month Dannielle and I moved into a split level, two bedroom, two bath apartment in Rota not far from the base. We had neighbors all around us and Dannielle could walk to the base or to the stores in Rota. Although Dannielle was 18 years old and had just graduated from high school, she didn't have a driver's license. Since the requirements for a foreigner to obtain a license were very strict as well as very expensive, we decided she would wait until our return to the states to get her driver's license. Dannielle had recently started working at the Navy Exchange on base and now she could set her own schedule instead of depending on me to take her and pick her up. I missed the pool, but this new apartment worked out much better.

Shortly before we were scheduled to leave Spain, I had a problem with Dannielle. I was at the office and received a call from the Spanish police at the on base air terminal telling me that Dannielle and an enlisted man were attempting to board a flight to Gibraltar. Well, you could have blown me over with a feather. I asked them to detain Dannielle and her friend until I got there which they were more than happy to do particularly since Dannielle's passport was issued by the Navy under my name and I had to accompany her when she used it. Dannielle was supposed to be at work at the Navy Exchange so this really caught me off guard. When I arrived at the terminal, I asked Dannielle and her traveling buddy Paul what was going on and she said they were going to elope to Gibraltar. The entire time we were talking, the two of them were looking down at the floor instead of at me. Dannielle knew she was in serious trouble and Paul acted like he was ready to bolt out of there. I could not believe this. These two knuckle heads actually thought they were going to elope. Dannielle was 19 years old now and in the states she could do what she wanted to do since she was considered an adult but not in Spain as my military dependent. Over the next few weeks I repeatedly asked her why she wanted to elope with Paul but I never got an answer. I finally decided that it was Dannielle's way of rebelling against me and telling me she was grown. This reminded me of when she used to say "I hate you, I want to go live with my father". This kid was living in Europe and wanted for nothing because her mom made very good money these days and she wanted to run off. Dannielle had grown up to be a very intelligent beautiful young lady who had her entire life in front of her. She could be anything she wanted to be, do anything she wanted to do, but running off to get married to a rag tail E-3 at the age of 19 would only force her into the life of "no pot, no window". I had struggled so hard all my life to get an education and rise above poverty in order for Dannielle to have a better life than I had. All the doors were open for her and she didn't even realize it. I fully expected Dannielle to go to college and consider a career in the military but I could only encourage her and hope she listened to my advice. None of this made much sense to me but it was obvious I could no longer trust Dannielle so I took her passport and locked it in my desk drawer at the office. Even though she wasn't allowed to travel without me, there was always the chance that the Spanish police at the civilian airport wouldn't know this and let her board a flight. Consequently, she also lost her job at the Navy Exchange since she didn't show up for work that day and the supervisor found out that she had tried to leave the country on my military passport. I never saw Paul again but heard a few weeks later that he had received transfer orders and had left Rota.

Unfortunately, my tour did not get extended to four years and before I knew it I had orders to return to the states for my twilight tour. I had really enjoyed working with NCIS and I hated to leave Spain. A twilight tour is the tour immediately prior to retirement and mine would be spent at Rickenbacker Air Base, Columbus, Ohio. Rickenbacker was a reserve training facility and I would spend my last eleven months on active duty as their Administrative Officer, Legal Officer, Training Officer and part time Security Officer. It isn't unusual for a naval officer to have numerous titles and responsibilities because one is primary and the others are secondary. My primary billet during this period was a training officer and I would be teaching and lecturing the drilling reservists. I was passed over for promotion to LCDR which wasn't a surprise to me because my tour with NCIS was not a promotable tour in the eyes of the Navy. In other words, it wasn't another tour at the Pentagon, or a tour on a ship, or a tour as an instructor at the Naval Academy. But I was alright with getting passed over and was looking forward to retirement at the early age of 42.

After a 15 hour return flight from Spain, Dannielle and I arrived in Columbus on the evening of December 13, 1992. It was very cold and snowing in Columbus when we landed and neither of us had a coat or boots. These are things you don't need in Spain. We checked into the Holiday Inn near the airport, got something to eat and went to bed. Dannielle and I had several cats in Spain and I decided to bring my favorite one, Blackie, back to the states with us. After that long flight, Blackie ate dinner, went to the litter box and then crashed in his cage until the next morning. I took a photo of him and Dannielle a couple of days later and I'm glad I did because he died the following year from what I assumed was a heart attack. Blackie was a beautiful but chunky solid black cat who we adopted from the Humane Society at Rota. He was really a great cat and I missed him for quite a while after he died. I haven't had another cat since.

The next morning, I called mom to tell her Dannielle and I had made it back to the states and were in Columbus. She was upset and told me that Ray had died of brain cancer the week prior while in the VA hospital in Dallas. I was shocked. I knew he had been sick but I had no idea he had brain cancer. Ray was the only stepfather I even half way liked because the two of them had been married for over ten years and he helped mom around the house the last few years since her diabetes had begun affecting her both physically and mentally. This was the beginning of the end for mom. Less than two years later it was necessary to sell her house and admit her to the nursing home in Athens where she subsequently died.

After talking to mom, I decided Dannielle and I needed to go shopping for some winter clothes but first I had to rent a car and find a shopping center. As it turned out, all the stores were now located in what was called a mall. There had been a lot of changes in the states while we were gone and the creation of malls was one of them. I rented a car from a rental agency located next to our hotel, got directions to the nearest mall, and Dannielle and I took off on our shopping spree. It was still snowing and I didn't have much experience driving in snow so the trip to the mall was quite perilous. We were slipping and sliding all over the road. I was only out in this mess because we needed coats, boots, some sweaters, and jeans. I was tired of freezing my butt off in this cold, snowy weather. Neither Dannielle nor I enjoyed our shopping experience at the mall. You had to park blocks away, walk that distance in the crappy weather, then wander around that ridiculous huge area looking for stores that sold clothes. And to top it off, there were hoards of people in the mall doing their Christmas shopping. I'm sorry, but I still prefer mom and pop stores or strip malls instead of this gigantic collection of stores that require you to walk until you are exhausted and fall out on one of the benches located in the middle of this monster. Whose cruel idea was this any way?

The following week I checked into Rickenbacker and found an apartment not far from the base. Our household goods and car arrived from Spain about three weeks later and Dannielle and I settled into our new apartment in a new city once again. During the next few months, Dannielle enrolled in college at Columbus State Community College but dropped out after one quarter. Then she enlisted in the Navy Reserves as a drilling reservist and made it through boot camp before becoming pregnant by some low life she had recently met. She was subsequently discharged from the Navy Reserves due to her pregnancy as well as her lack of drill participation and eventually married then divorced David, the low life. As a matter of fact, I paid for their divorce in 1995 because

Dannielle was now a single parent and couldn't afford it. I had hoped my daughter would take advantage of the opportunities I had created for her but she chose not to. Like Big Momma used to say "you can lead a horse to the water trough but you can't make him drink". I completed my eleven month twilight tour at Rickenbacker and retired from the Navy on November 1, 1993, with slightly over 21 years of active duty service. My retirement from the Navy put me one step closer to avoiding the "no pot, no window" syndrome in the years to come.

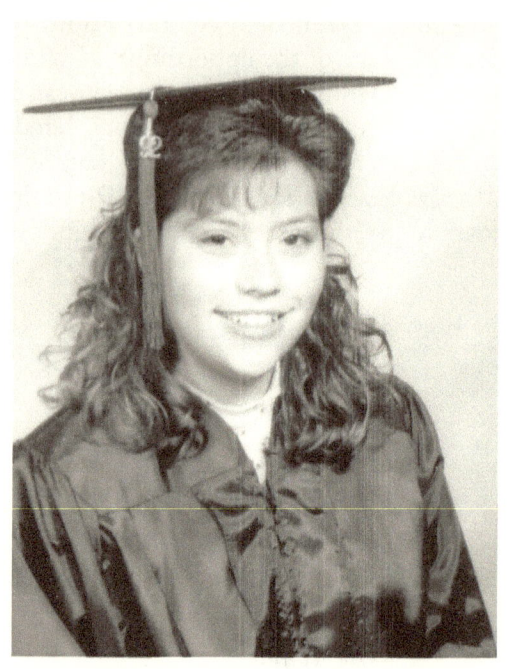

Dannielle, High School Graduation, 1992

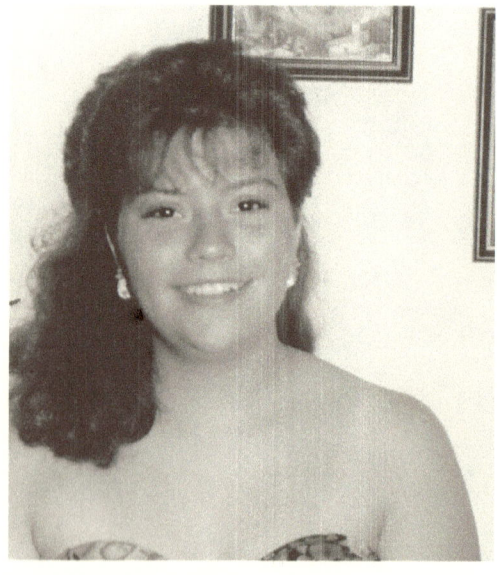

Dannielle's prom photo, 1991

CHAPTER 10

Conclusion

I have often said that my life reads like a Shakespearian Tragedy and after reading this novel I am sure you agree. I had the misfortune of being born into a life of poverty to parents with very little education or motivation. My alcoholic, abusive father abandoned us when I was a child and my co-dependent mother was absent from my life for many years. After my father abandoned us, my mother was focused primarily on marrying into money instead of raising her three children. She was married nine times (twice to the same man) and never found her Prince Charming, just one ugly frog after another. Since she never found a rich husband to support her and she didn't like to work, my mother quit working at the age of 55 and starting drawing social security disability. Consequently, the taxpayers supported her for twenty years until she died penniless in a nursing home at the age of 75. When I was ten years old, my mother sent my two sisters and me to live with my maternal grandparents for three years. Since they did not want the responsibility of raising us either, I always felt unloved, unwanted and a burden on them. At the age of 16, I was forced to get a job and for the lack of other options, began supporting myself. At the height of the Viet Nam War, with my mother's consent, I joined the United States Air Force at the age of 17, and after some bumps in the road began the long process of improving my life. I was married and divorced three times before the age of 30, resulting in me becoming a single parent to my only child, Dannielle, when she was two years old. Through my bad judgment, my first two husbands had the same disgusting unacceptable traits as my father. My first husband was an abusive alcoholic and my second husband abandoned his family, Dannielle and I, for a new Chevy SS his parents bought him as enticement to throw us out on the street. Unfortunately, too many parents (usually men) walk away from their parental responsibility thereby creating a financial hardship for the single parent. A child needs the influence, love, and financial support of both parents in their lives and a child support check does not fulfill their parental responsibility. Additionally, at the age of 32, I was diagnosed with Stage II breast cancer and underwent a radical mastectomy, chemotherapy, and several reconstructive surgeries. Fortunately, I survived breast cancer and am still cancer free 26 years later, but the five year struggle to recover mentally, physically, and financially was horrendous. Through perseverance, hard work, sheer determination and most importantly education, I changed my life. Education, preferably a college degree, is empowering and offers opportunities that would not otherwise be available. I refused to accept the pathetic life of "no pot, no window" to which I was born. I obtained a Bachelor of Arts degree in 1982 from the University of Mississippi and a Masters of Forensic Science from George Washington University in 1986. After serving my country for 21 years, I retired as a Lieutenant from the United States Navy at the age of 42. No one is immune from the "no pot, no window" syndrome but everyone has the ability to overcome it. This is the year 2010, and I have had many life challenges since my retirement from the Navy in 1993, but I was always able to overcome them. This was possible only because of my higher education level and my service and subsequent retirement from the military. While recovering from breast cancer, I made a vow to live the rest of my life with no regrets. To date, I have only one regret and that is my daughter and I do not and have not had a close relationship since she left home at the age of 19. Apparently my required absences during Dannielle's childhood as well as my sending her to live briefly with her father and my mother while I was receiving treatment for breast cancer caused her to distance herself from me. Hopefully, my life is far from over and our relationship will improve. I have shared my life story in hopes that it has motivated and inspired all of you with similar family histories and/ or circumstances to pull yourselves out of the abyss of the "no pot, no window" syndrome and strive to change your sour lemons to sweet lemonade as well. We all have the ability to create our destinies and thank goodness anything is possible. Good Luck!

Final Thoughts

THROUGH THE EYES OF A CHILD

A short story contributed by my sister, Anne Evans

My daddy wants to ask you to hold his hand, to have faith to believe and trust in Him, and to accept His unconditional love and blessings that He has for each one of us. As a little child, grab hold of His hand and never let go.

I would like to dedicate this book to my children and grandchildren so that they are able to understand the love of God that was shown to me causing a life change in my life that would cause my descendants to have a new future, a new heritage, breaking the power of many strongholds and generational curses off of them. "My Father holds the universe in his hands and I am his child."

When I was eight years old and very much of a daddy's girl, my whole life changed. Daddy left us and moved to a different city many miles away, Baytown, and later Houston. He visited the family on an average of maybe three times a year until I was fourteen years old when he disappeared out of our lives. It was at that time that Mom and Dad got a divorce. I did not understand what had happened and no one talked to me about what had happened. I missed my daddy very much. We went fishing, frog gigging, riding on the family horse Snowball, and at times just sat on the back steps together. It was on the back steps that I learned from Daddy how to tie my shoes and how to whistle. Some of my favorite times that we spent together were on Red River where we went fishing, frog gigging, and camping. I missed the good times but not the bad times when I was afraid for myself and sisters because Daddy was drunk and in a drunken rage.

Mom had always been distant to my sisters and me and seemed to try to get rid of us all the time instead of wanting us to be around her. The only time that I was asked to be with her was if she wanted her hair brushed, her nails painted, or her eyebrows plucked. Mom would lock us out of the house with a jar of water to play all day outside until supper time. Then she would be able to sleep, listen to the radio, talk on the phone, and watch TV. We had nothing outside to play with and had to use our imagination. We would go through the trash getting out things such as aluminum pie plates to make chocolate pies made of dirt or an oatmeal container to collect pretty rocks or insects. We would play house. If you had to use the bathroom then you had to use it on the ground with no toilet paper. My sisters, Mary and Betty, were four and five years respectively younger than I. After my parents separated, at eight years old I was made to be in charge of the care of my sisters and the house. I was to walk my sisters to school or to our great aunt's house down the block before I left for school, prepare something to eat for us in the evening, get my sisters and self ready for bed with baths for everyone, and make our lunch putting them in brown bags in the refrigerator for morning. When my sisters were in bed, then it was time to pick up the house, wash the dishes, wash clothes that we needed in the bathtub and let drip dry, and get my homework. Some of the worst spankings that I ever received from Mom was because the house was not picked up or because I did not make all A's on my report card. Because I did make A's I was promoted to the accelerated class taking classes that were two years ahead of others in the same grade. It was so hard that at the age of fourteen our family doctor said that my nerves needed a rest. I went to live with my maternal grandparents and stayed until I graduated from high school and left with a scholarship to attend junior college. I finally got to be a kid at the age of fourteen and it was so much fun! Big Daddy and Big Momma, Joe and Cora McCormack, lived in Elysian Fields, Texas. Elysian Fields is a very small town on the county line of Texas and Louisiana. Big Daddy owned a service station. He let me earn extra money by gassing up cars and trucks, checking the oil, and washing the windshields. I loved my job and looked the part dressed in jeans with a red rag hanging out of my back jean pocket. He also had an icehouse at the station. I was allowed to get the blocks of ice out for the customer, which was also fun. At the station, there were cookies the size of a dinner plate in a big jar for a nickel. There were Dr. Peppers and ice-cream sandwiches that never ran out. It was a great place for a kid and I was earning spending money! Then I became sixteen! All of the boys liked the way I looked, I think, because I became popular with the boys! I joined the band playing the French horn, played on the basketball team as guard, was the art editor for the school paper, was a four year member of the Honor Roll Society, and my senior year was elected cheerleader. In my high school years I started smoking and later drinking hard liquor. I got a fake ID that the kids at school were making for a price and went with other kids that liked to drink to the Strip in Bossier City using our fake ID's. The ID's allowed us to get into any dance hall that we tried and to order as many drinks as we could afford. I liked going to the Strip to drink and dance when James Brown was singing and playing his saxophone. You ask how did I get to do that and be allowed to live in my grandparent's house. At night before I came in the house for supper and a bath I would take the screen off of my bedroom window, crawl in the window putting the screen under my bed, and then go back out the window coming in the door. Then when my grandparents were asleep I could crawl out the window and meet the kids in a car parked on the road waiting. When I came back, I crawled in the window, put the screen back on, and went to bed. It worked for a long time until I started getting really drunk, forgot, and came through the front door waking them up and smelling like a brewery with Jack Daniels or Jim Beam. I was grounded in what seemed like forever. Another time that I was grounded forever was when I hid behind the back school bus seat not getting off at school and then hitch hiking to Bossier when the bus driver parked the bus and left. I spent the whole day in Bossier at the movies and window-shopping hitch hiking all the way. All of this so far sounds pretty normal for a teenager, but there was nothing normal about what had happened in my life before I went to live with my grandparents.

When I was eight years old my parents starting arguing and physically fighting almost all of the time. The domestic violence was terrifying to me as a child. I understood that they did not like each other much less love each other and became afraid that one would hurt the other one really bad or hurt me and my sisters. If Dad was drunk, would he physically hurt us, his children, or would he try to take us with him to where he lived? If Mom tried to leave in the car when they were arguing, he would chase us in his truck. Once he shot the back car window out and I was sitting on the back seat. Before he actually hit the window, I had balled up on the floor board with my head covered by my arms. Then there was the time that he came to my bedroom window with a rifle asking me to let him in the house. He said that he was going to shoot that Bitch meaning Mom. I ran out of the bedroom only to find him standing in the dark looking through Mom's bedroom window when she was sleeping. I woke her up and she called the police. He left immediately. There was the time that I woke up because I heard crying and screaming. I went into the dining room half asleep to find Mom sliding down the wall crying hysterically with Dad holding a hunting knife to her throat as she slid down. I think that he found out that she was dating. She got loose and ran out of the house and off in her car. We were left there in the house with him. I hid in the closet or played like I was sleeping when there were times like this. I tried and tried in my mind to understand and plan how I would get out of the house if needed with my two sisters and where we would go. It was scary because the trauma usually happened at night and I was afraid of the dark. Many times after Dad left and moved away Mom would not come home at night. It was very scary for me thinking that someone might break into our house. I couldn't sleep. We did not have air conditioning and had only one fan that had to stay in Mom's room. Therefore, the windows were always up when it was hot outdoors. Anyone could get the screen off or cut through it and get in the house. At the age of 40 years old plus, Jesus delivered me from the feeling and fear of abandonment. I was moving in the line with my tray at a cafeteria getting my food when I realized that Jesus was standing on my right side and moving with me in line. When I acknowledged him, He said to me to remember back when I was young and was in the house with my sisters at night all alone and afraid. He said that I was to feel not afraid because He was with me and watching over us. Jesus asked me to visualize Him with me in the house so that I could see in my mind's eye that He was with me. When I saw in my mind that Jesus had been there all the time, the fear of abandonment left.

Mom in total married nine times, twice to one man. Dad married eight times. It is hard for anyone to imagine that a child would have seventeen different parent figures or adults telling you what to do. Some of the men that Mom was in a relationship with chased us or tried to corner us for sex. We would then have to leave the house going anywhere that we could until Mom returned home. Dad dated and had relationships with women that had substance abuse problems or had been raised in a night club environment. The fighting between the two, Dad and his woman, continued because both were under the influence of a substance. If I went to visit my dad, he would wake me up during the middle of the night threatening to spank me if I didn't cook him something to eat and then sit and listen to him sing a song in his drunken voice. I was always very small in size. I would stand on a chair and cut up potatoes for French fries and then move the chair to the stove to put the fries in hot grease to fry them. Looking back, that was so dangerous for a child eight years old. I was spanked with a belt or with a wire fly swatter. Both left whelps and cut the skin leaving bruises. The whelps would ooze and stick to my clothes and the sheet causing the healing to be slow. The worst spanking that I got was from my mom because I did not make all A's on my report card. I was spanked with a belt with the buckle hitting me. The buckle had teeth that grabbed my skin and cut. I had to get behind the commode to protect myself from being beaten. I was the oldest child and the one that looked like my dad. Mom was not emotionally stable we discovered when we three children grew up. Once she set the house on fire that she lived in because she wanted to leave her current husband and collect the insurance money at the same time. Because gasoline was poured around the house and then set on fire, for some reason not known to me, her husband went to prison for arson.

When my maternal grandparents died, I felt all alone and that no one really cared because there was no family left. My sisters had since turned against me because they said that I was the one that was rescued from the hell that we lived in and got special privileges by living in the care of my grandparents. I had lost contact with my dad and did not know how to locate him. I did not know if he was even alive. Mom went to live permanently in a nursing home when she was 55 years old. She died in a nursing home at the age of 75. She lived twenty years in a nursing home because there was no one willing or wanting to care for her and have her live in their home.

Because I felt that no one really cared or loved me, I decided that it did not matter what I did in life or even if I lived. With that mind set and attitude I met a very handsome man that was an emergency medical technician but was as wild as a March hare when he was not in uniform working. He liked loud music, marijuana, beer, fast cars and motorcycles, and just a wild time. We would go on motorcycle rides after midnight half naked and half under the influence and would be going a speed over 80 and up to 100 miles/hour. Of course, no one was properly dressed to ride a motorcycle and wore no helmet. We were an accident waiting to happen. We would ride with other couples in the same shape as we were and same mind set and would stop wherever we thought we would be comfortable or it seemed romantic. Life was good and we later married. This continued on until I became sick with hepatitis and was out of work for three and half months. Then when I got back on my feet and back to work, I became pregnant. After having the baby, my second child, I had to have a hysterectomy ten months later due to my uterus pulling from the muscles during child birth. The doctor had tried to repair my uterus in surgery after child birth, but I continued to hemorrhage for 10 months after child birth and surgery. The traumas and having to care for two children separated my husband and me in our relationship since we did not have time for each other anymore. A year and half later after the birth of our daughter, my husband decided to start using hard drugs again shooting up speed and cocaine. I did not know that he had used hard drugs in high school. It was all a nightmare to me and left me to believe that I had the responsibility of raising two children by myself. He had not gone back to college when I had hepatitis because he said that he needed to work. But when he started to use hard drugs, he was working full time at a car wash. We had little money and our financial responsibilities were suffering.

It was a year or so after he started to use hard drugs again that he seemed to be loosing his sense of reality. It was not long after that time that he was holding us captive in our mobile home. He had nailed all of the windows closed from the outside and put a log chain around the length of the trailer when he would leave locking us in the trailer. My fairly new 1968 Camaro was stripped of all electrical wiring, jacked up with the tires and rims taken off and missing so that I could not drive the car or have someone tow it for repairs. My children and I were prisoners in our own home. The home phone line on the outside pole was cut by him. Since we lived in a pasture away from neighbors and the main road, it was hard for me to try to think who would stop and help us even if I did get out of the trailer with both children. The trailer was parked in the pasture with the cows that all belonged to my in laws. They turned their heads and tried not to think or interfere in whatever was or seemed to be happening at the trailer. When he was home, he made us all get down and hide when a car was heard or an airplane or helicopter was heard going over the house. My husband said that the Mafia was coming to get us and that we would be kidnapped and killed. He kept guns loaded and propped at the windows and doors. A shoulder holster that he wore carried a 357 Magnum. At night, he would walk around playing with and spinning the 357. He would come to my bed and spin the barrel of the 357 in my ear. Shortly after my husband starting using hard drugs when my baby girl was approximately 1 and half years old and my son was 7 years old, my husband was institutionalized at a state mental hospital due to paranoid schizophrenia with delusions. He was still using hard drugs and abusing alcohol at the time, so the evaluation stated that the schizophrenia, paranoia, delusions, etc. could have been brought on by the abuse of drugs, alcohol, and stress. I constantly fought the thoughts of him being released and killing all of us and possibly himself. After evaluations, tests, counseling, and medication administered to my husband to keep the paranoia and delusions in check, he was released as an out patient with Mental Health and Retardation with the understanding that appointments would be made by him for weekly counseling and medication checks. Six months after his release from the mental hospital he shot the side of his face off with the 357 committing suicide when the children and I were gone to buy groceries. You ask, how can a person many years later still be in their right mind typing this? The answer lies in God being with me all of the time even if I didn't know it or feel His presence. After identifying my husband and making funeral arrangements at the morgue, I went outside where it was dark with only light from the stars and moon as I looked up in the sky. I cried out to God to help me. All of my life I had tried to survive. Now I had two children to raise alone with no job, home, automobile, savings, and no support. I also had the expense of a funeral and headstone. I was so angry that my husband had left me in such a situation because it seemed that he was only thinking of himself. God heard my cry and had been waiting all of the time for me to ask Him for help. He is waiting for all of us to ask for His help so that He has permission to be involved in our lives. My life has never been the same since that moment. I felt His unconditional love, I felt the love and sacrifice that Jesus had for me, and I felt the comfort and encouragement from the Holy Spirit at that time and then from then on. God empowered me with the filling of the Holy Spirit giving me the hope and boldness that was needed to go on in life and to overcome. God has repeatedly given to me, loved me unconditionally, and met every need that I have had. He is always on time and has never failed. All that He asked of us is to come to Him as a little child believing that He can and will take care of us in every way if we have faith to believe. God is our Daddy and Jesus is our big brother. Nothing is impossible if God is for you and not against you.

I'm writing this to encourage those of you who say or think that life has really dealt them a bad hand and that they are not responsible for the life and the decisions that they have made causing them to fail blaming God, their parents, circumstances, situations, etc. There is so much that I could not cognitively understand as a child, and so much that I blocked out because of the pain and hurt. I lived in fear and did not have hope of a future or that it would get any better. In the book of Jeremiah, the word says that "God has a plan for each one of us and that it is for our good and not evil and to give us a hope and a future". My daddy wants to ask you to hold his hand, to have faith to believe and trust in Him, and to accept His unconditional love and blessings that He has for each one of us. As a little child, grab hold of His hand and never let go. The blessings of Abraham, eternal life, peace, restoration, deliverance, and healing are all given to us freely as a gift from Jesus paid with the price of His own life as He was humiliated, tortured, mocked, and then killed for us. With the resurrection power of his father, God, Jesus was raised from the dead conquering death and hell and sits at the right hand of God making intercession for us always. He loves us unconditionally and gave everything for our redemption and our restoration back into fellowship with God, our creator and Daddy. I can blame my parents for the bad choices that I made in life, I can blame my husband for hardships when he made the choice to commit suicide, I can choose to hold unforgiveness towards them, and I can go on through life feeling defeated and cheated out of many things. But I chose to ask God for His help and to have faith to believe that He loves me unconditionally and knows as my dad what is best for me. Accept His love, accept the free gift that Jesus gave to us and that our father sacrificed for us, and come to Him. His arms are open to us always. The word says in the book of Isaiah that "His ear is not deaf that He can not hear our cry or His arm too short that He can not reach out and save us". Run to Him! He loves us unconditionally!

—